AF573953

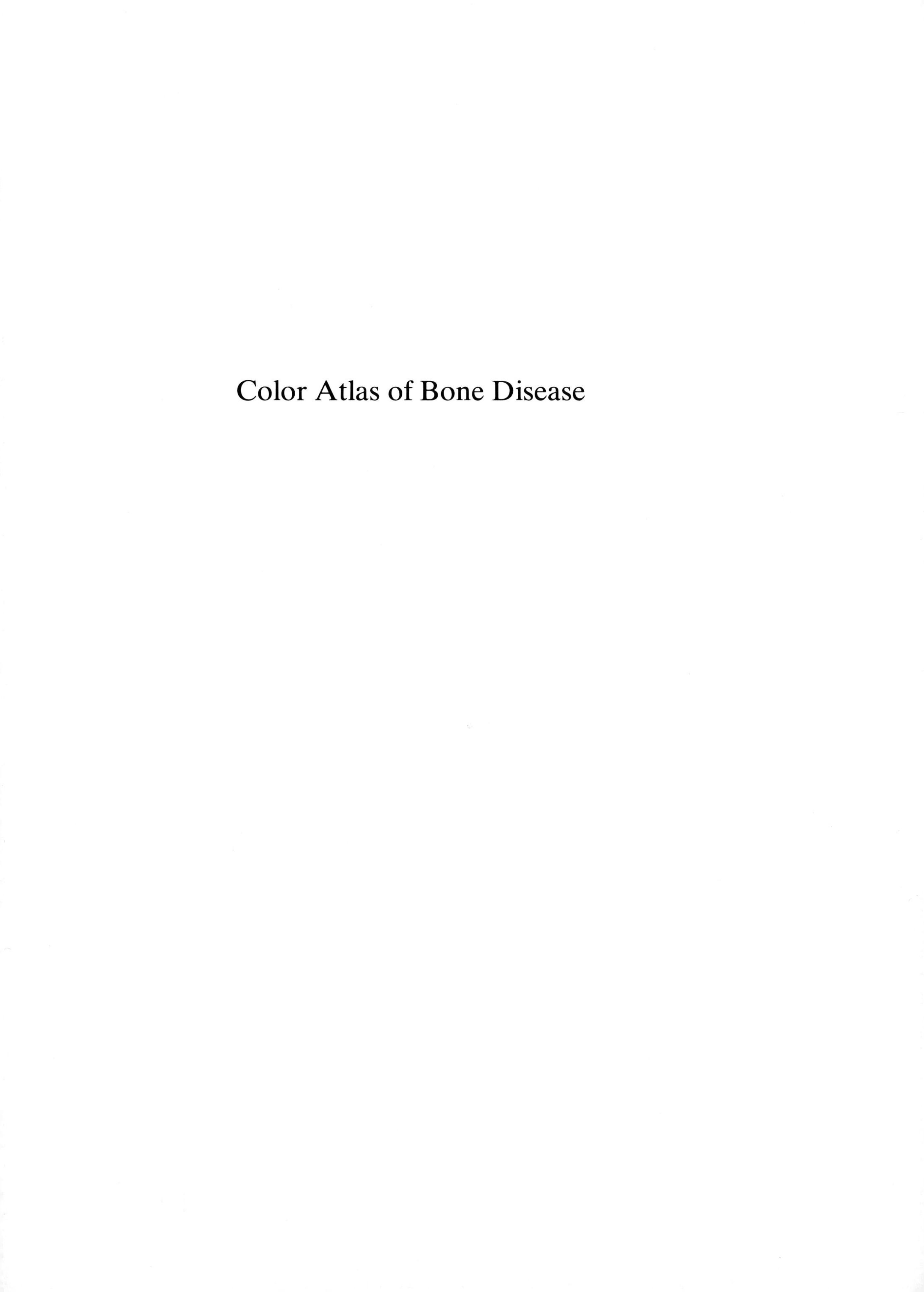

Color Atlas of Bone Disease

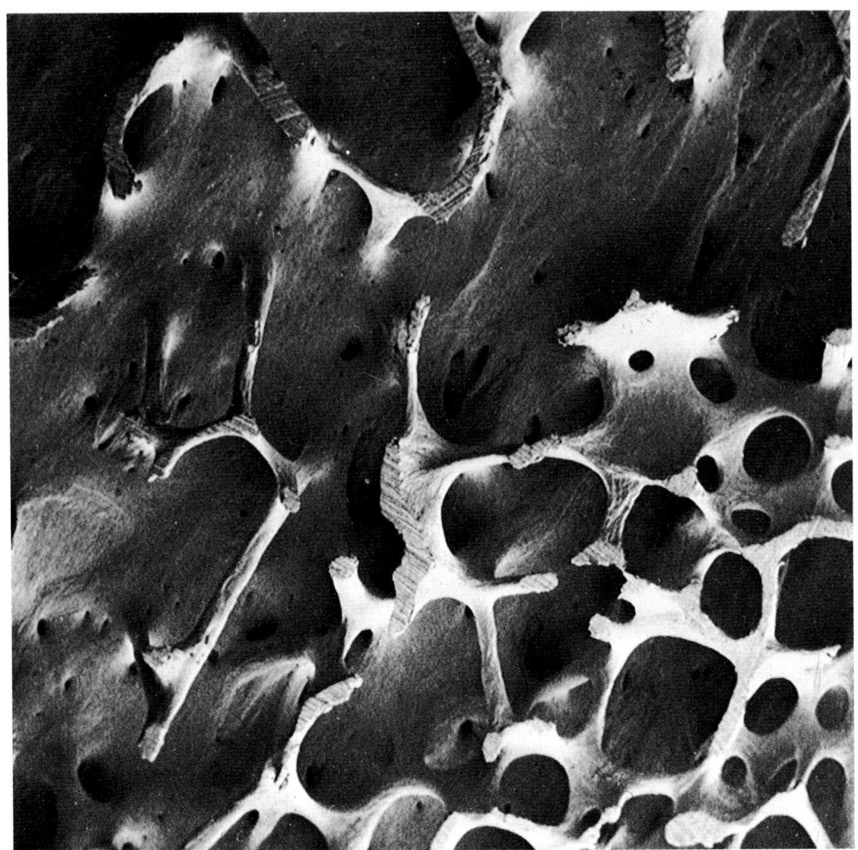

Cancellous bone structure

Color Atlas of Bone Disease

Victor Parsons
DM FRCP

Physician, King's College Hospital
and Renal Unit, Dulwich Hospital
formerly Senior Lecturer in Medicine
King's College Hospital, University of London

Year Book Medical Publishers, Inc
35 East Wacker Drive, Chicago

Distributed in Continental North, South and Central America,
Hawaii, Puerto Rico and the Philippines by
Year Book Medical Publishers, Inc.
By arrangement with Wolfe Medical Publications Ltd.
Printed by Smeets-Weert, Holland

Library of Congress Cataloging in Publication Data
Parsons, Victor.
Color atlas of bone disease.

Includes index.
1. Bones – Diseases. I. Title.
RC930.P37 616.7′1′00222 79-23922
ISBN 0-8151-6635-4

Series Editor (Medical): G. Barry Carruthers, MD(Lond)

Other books in these series (Medical, Surgical)
already published:
Color Atlas of General Pathology
Color Atlas of Ophthalmological Diagnosis
Color Atlas of Renal Diseases
Color Atlas of Venereology
Color Atlas of Dermatology
Color Atlas of Infectious Diseases
Color Atlas of Ear, Nose & Throat Diagnosis
Color Atlas of Rheumatology
Color Atlas of Microbiology
Color Atlas of Forensic Pathology
Color Atlas of Pediatrics
Color Atlas of Histology
Color Atlas of General Surgical Diagnosis
Color Atlas of Physical Signs in General Medicine
Color Atlas of Tropical Medicine & Parasitology
Color Atlas of Human Anatomy
Color Atlas of Cardiac Pathology
Color Atlas of Histological Staining Techniques
Atlas of Cardiology: ECGs and Chest X-Rays
Color Atlas of Neuropathology
Color Atlas of Gynecological Surgery
(Volumes 1–3; Volumes 4–6 in preparation)
Color Atlas of Liver Disease
Post-Mortem Procedures (An illustrated textbook)
Color Atlas of Endocrinology
Color Atlas of Ocular Tumors
Color Atlas of Pathogenic Fungi
Color Atlas of Temporal Bone Surgical Anatomy
Color Atlas of Tumor Histopathology
Color Atlas of Diabetes
Color Atlas of Peripheral Vascular Diseases
Color Atlas of Clinical Orthopaedics

Contents

Preface

Bone disease is uniquely investigated by a good history, clinical examination and appropriate radiology. The majority of traumatic, inflammatory and neoplastic diseases are quickly recognised and further investigation is not often carried out. Metabolic and endocrine bone disease is detected by simple blood tests and in this way most physicians and surgeons diagnose the disease and initiate treatment. This book illustrates the mechanisms at the cellular and microscopic level of these disease processes; the number of radiographs and comment on biochemical findings is therefore kept to a minimum. Tissue biopsy has led to an understanding of the different types of bone disease underlying trauma and neoplastic and metabolic disease. I hope that the common disease processes are well represented; a few rarer diseases are also described to show underlying processes. A bibliography is included to encourage further reading as it is not the purpose of this short illustrated atlas to provide the detail and discussion found in longer texts.

The magnifications of histology pictures refer to the original 35 mm transparencies.

Acknowledgements

I am grateful to my colleagues in the Orthopaedic Department, Mr R. Crellin, Mr C. Holden, Mr T. Morley and Mr M. Thomas, for their generous referral of many patients illustrated here. Drs E. Hamilton, H. Berry and J. Goodwill (Rheumatologists) have provided a range of diagnostic problems, many of which are included here. Dr John Laws and Dr Heather Nunnerley have been responsible for the choice of several radiographs, Dr John Barratt for the isotope scans and Dr Alan Darby for some of the bone histology.

I am indebted to Ms Siew Bazany and Mr John Blewitt of the Medical Illustration Department, to Mr William Brackenbury, who prepared many of the illustrations, and to Mrs Penny Leach, Mrs Pat Niblett and Ms Penny Lock for secretarial help.

I should also like to thank the many colleagues listed below for their generous help over the years and for the loan of illustrations:

Professor A. Boyd and S. Jones (**86**, **108**), Dr A. C. Boyle (**321**, from *A Colour Atlas of Rheumatology*, Wolfe Medical Publications Ltd), Dr M. Dynski-Klein (**281**, **284**, from *A Colour Atlas of Paediatrics*, Wolfe Medical Publications Ltd), Professor J. Garret, Dr P. Gishen (**75**), Dr Haji Haroon, Professor M. Harris and Professor Gerald Winter, Eastman Dental Hospital, London (**2**, **3**, **4**, **180**), Dr J. Jowsey (**62**, **87**, **94**, **135**, **136**), Dr M. Kataria (**164**), Professor D. N. S. Kerr (**5**), Professor Ata Khan, Professor S. M. Krane and Professor C. Nagant (**123**, **124**), Dr G. Levene (**20**, from *A Colour Atlas of Dermatology*, Wolfe Medical Publications Ltd), Dr Andrew MacFarlane, Dr William Marshall (**268**, **269**), Dr A. Mowatt (**57**), Professor B. E. C. Nordin (**80**), Dr C. R. Paterson (**9**, **47**, **285**), Dr Munro Peacock and Editors of *Medicine* (**26**, **60**, **171**, first published in: Peacock, M., Endocrine Control of Calcium and Phosphorus Metabolism, *Medicine*, 1978, *Endocrine Diseases*, series 3, volume 9, page 407), Dr Keith Pettingale (**294**, **295**), Dr Brian Preston, Mr B. C. O'Riordan (**191**, **192**), Professor P. Rubin and Year Book Medical Publishers Inc. (**331**, **332**, reproduced with permission from Rubin, P.: *Dynamic Classification of Bone Dysplasias*. Copyright © 1964 by Year Book Medical Publishers Inc., Chicago), Professor Khalil Salman, Professor W. Sandritter and F. K. Schattauer Verlag, Stuttgart (**208**, **212**, **231**, **241**, **247**, **276**, **293**, modified from illustrations in *Colour Atlas and Textbook of Macropathology*), Professor J. Sela (**86**), Professor H. Sissons (**142**, **143**), Dr R. Smith (**70**, **285**), Professor H. de Wardener and Dr John Eastwood, Department of Medicine, Charing Cross Hospital Medical School, London (**26**, **54**), Professor R. Warwick, Professor Peter Williams and Mr Richard Moore, Illustrator, Guy's Hospital (**95**, reproduced from figure 3.10, page 217 of 35th edition of *Gray's Anatomy*, Churchill Livingstone, 1973), Dr W. J. Whitehouse (frontispiece), Williams and Williams Publishers: Albright and Reifenstein, *Parathyroid Glands and Bone Disease* (**76**), Dr N. Woodhouse (**63**, **160**).

To compose an atlas of bone disease without the constant stimulus and advice of a morbid anatomist would be impossible, and I am greatly indebted to Professor George Stirling, MD, FRCPath, Professor of Pathology, King Abdulaziz University, Jeddah (formerly Reader in Pathology, University of Nottingham), whose help throughout the preparation of this book has been invaluable.

1. Introduction: Presentation and history

Bone forms part of the supporting tissues of the body and shares many of the disorders of these tissues. Because of the large number of disciplines involved, bone abnormalities do not 'belong' to one group of specialists but are shared between several specialities. It is hoped that this book will increase interest in skeletal disorders so that communication between specialists is improved to the benefit of the patient.

To be aware of the help that can be obtained from each discipline, it is necessary to use a variety of investigational techniques to determine the cause of the symptoms. The chief symptoms are pain, swelling, stiffness of joints, deformity and weakness. This emphasises immediately the links between primary care physicians, general surgeons, radiologists and other specialists as shown in the table below.

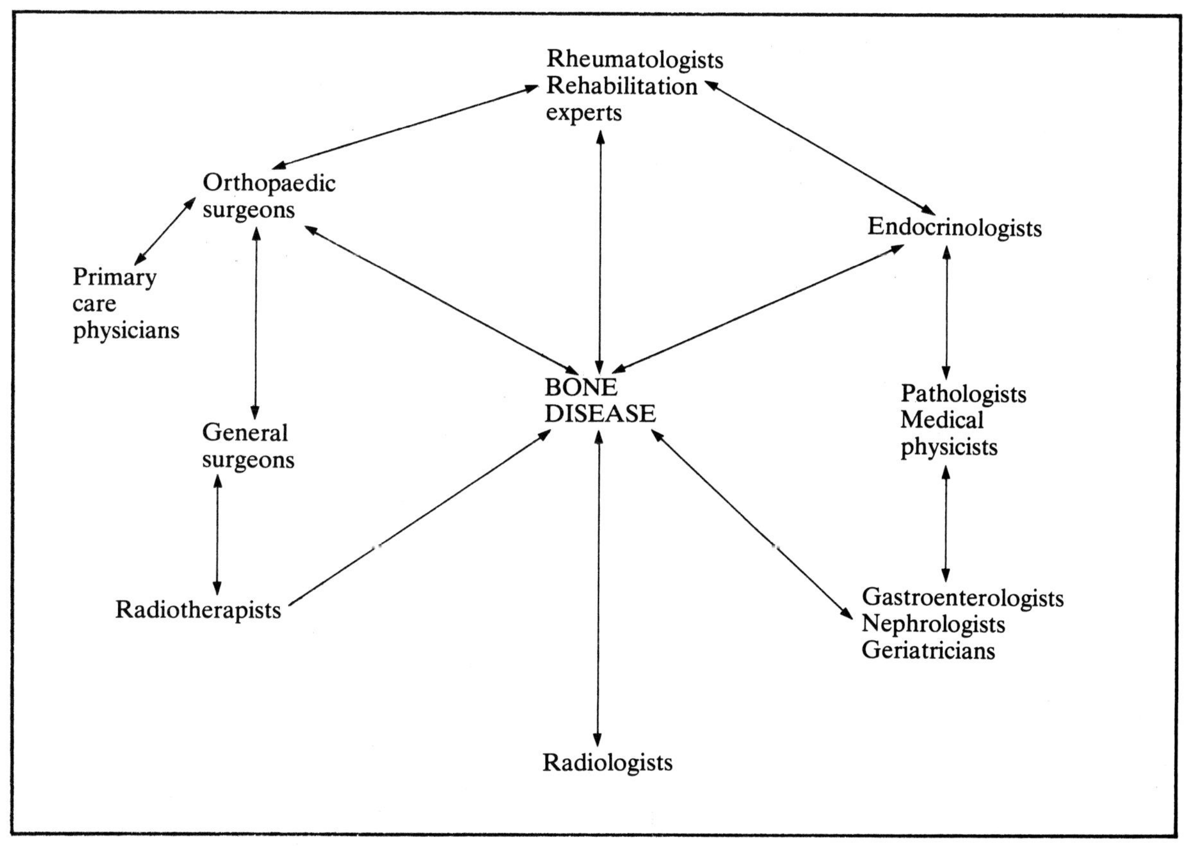

The clinical history of a patient with suspected bone disease should be taken with the aim of discovering some of the pathological mechanisms behind the symptoms of pain, deformity, muscle weakness, joint involvement and possible fracture.

Certain fundamental requirements must be met for the adequate functioning of bone:

- an adequate supply of matrix and mineral materials
- a normal luminal and transport function of the gut
- a bone cell population that is capable of synthesis and turnover
- correct hormonal balance matching formation and resorption
- sufficient physical stress across and within bone
- a freedom from invasion or involvement with other disease

Each part of the history, examination and investigation looks at these facets in turn.

a. Nutritional history and drug ingestion

The intake of calcium, phosphate, magnesium, other minerals and vitamin D should be enquired into when taking the history. The following tables illustrate the nutritional value of some common foods. See Appendix on page 104 for illustrations.

1. High calcium foods

	mg/100g
Dried potato	1702
Skimmed milk	1265
Cheese	810
Spinach	595
Sardines	409
Raw dried figs	284
Milk drink	274
Milk chocolate	246
Broccoli	160
White bread	100

2. High phosphate foods

	mg/100g
Meat extract	3200
Dried skimmed milk	1050
Cocoa	852
Bran	815
Sardines	683
Liver	576
Cheese	545
Egg yolk	495
Smoked fish	426
Peanuts	365

3. Vitamin content of food

Vitamin D containing foods

	Vit D IU/100 g	μg
Cod liver oil	8,700	217.5
Raw kippers	900	22.5
Margarine	300	7.5
Canned sardines	300	7.5
Whole raw eggs	70	1.75
Butter	40	1.0
Double cream (S)	20	0.5
Double cream (W)	7	0.175
Milk (S)	1.5	0.038
Milk (W)	0.5	0.013

(Conversion based on 40 IU = 1 μg)
(S = summer W = winter)

High vitamin C foods

	Vit C mg/kg
Rose hip syrup	150
Stewed blackcurrants	140
Raw cabbage	60
Fresh strawberries	60
Oranges	50
Grapefruit juice	35
New potatoes	30
Fried liver	20
Cooked cabbage	20
Fresh tomatoes	20

Drug induced bone disease

Bone disease can be the result of the ingestion of drugs and toxic materials which should be enquired into, for example:

- steroids, (**1**) a patient on steroids for protracted asthma showing facial plethora
- anticonvulsant induced bone disease, (**2**) a patient on anticonvulsants showing gum hypertrophy
- demineralisation is associated with
  - aluminium hydroxide and alkalis in excess
  - vitamin D as a tonic
  - prolonged heparin for anticoagulation
  - thyroxine for slimming
- tetracycline causing staining of the teeth (**3**), and bones

1 Steroid ingestion

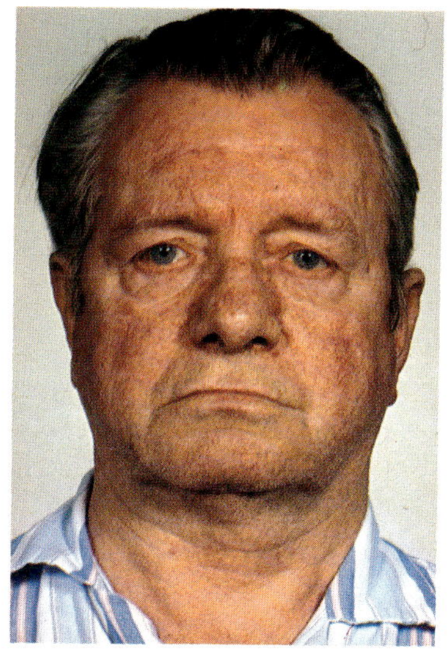

2 Anticonvulsant induced bone disease

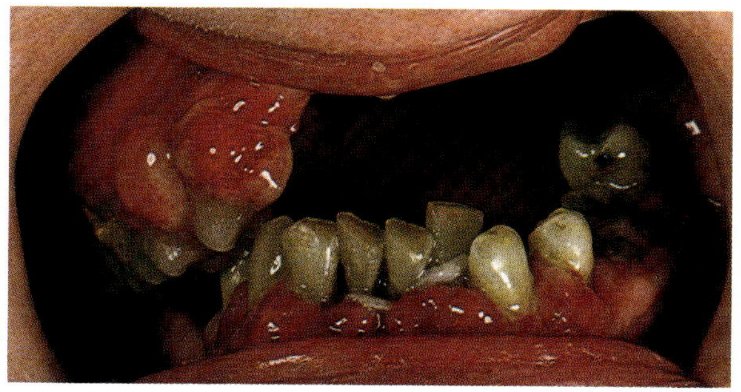

3 Tetracycline staining

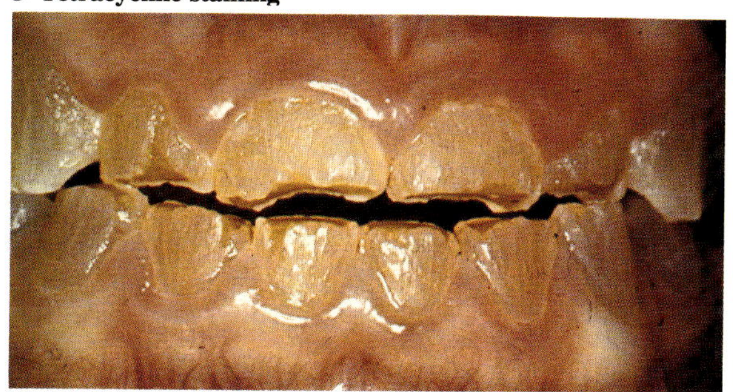

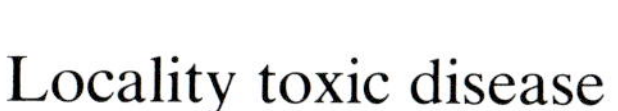

Locality toxic disease

- fluorosis, near factories processing aluminium, causing mottling of teeth (**4**) and affecting bones
- Itai Itai disease (Minamata disease), from the ingestion of fish contaminated by cadmium from a battery factory in Minamata Bay, Japan, causing bone pain
- 'Newcastle' dialysis bone disease, from dialysis against water treated with aluminium-containing salts, (**5**) showing gross myopathy

5 Newcastle dialysis bone disease

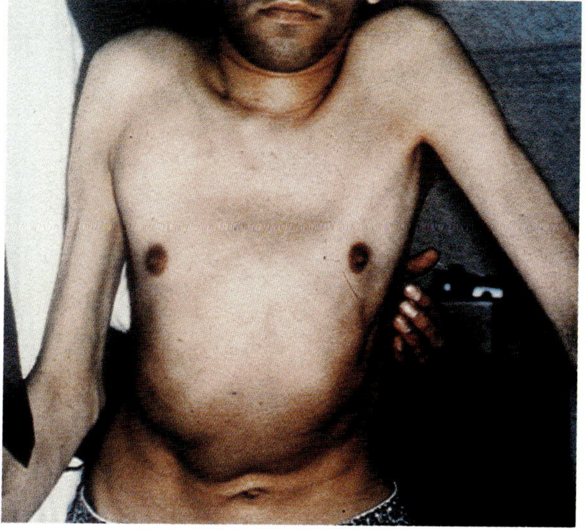

4 Fluorotic mottling of teeth

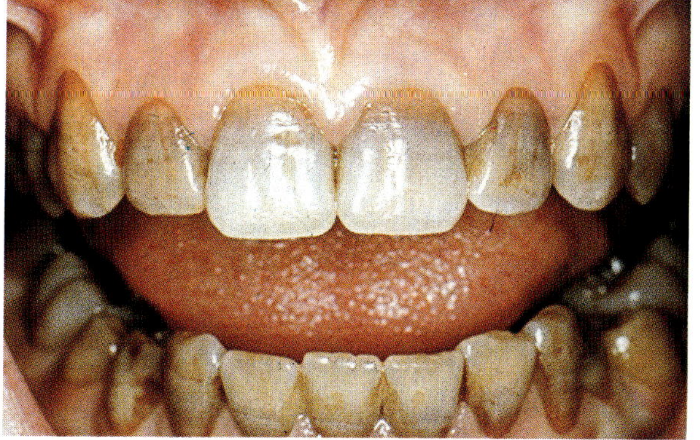

b. Past history

A brief enquiry should then be made into illnesses affecting the absorption and distribution of the elements which are essential for bone structure.

1. Achlorhydria – gastric surgery, (**6**) a radiograph of the stomach and gut showing intestinal hurry
2. Hepatic dysfunction – cirrhosis and osteoporosis (**7**) in a man with the Budd-Chiari syndrome
3. Pancreatic failure – steatorrhoea (fibrocystic disease of the pancreas), (**8**) a post-mortem pancreas from a girl who died in her late teens
4. Small bowel disorders
   - diverticulae
   - coeliac disease (before change of diet) showing severe stunting of growth, (**9**) this 58 year old woman is 1.37 m tall
   - Crohn's disease
   - fistula formation
5. Operations – short circuits and resection
6. Lactose-sensitivity, due to lactase deficiency A barium meal with 50 g of sucrose shows a normal pattern (**10**). When lactose is substituted the pattern is broken up (**11**). The handling of dietary and endogenous calcium in the gut is shown in **12**; with malabsorption output can exceed intake causing a negative calcium balance.

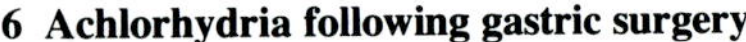

6 Achlorhydria following gastric surgery

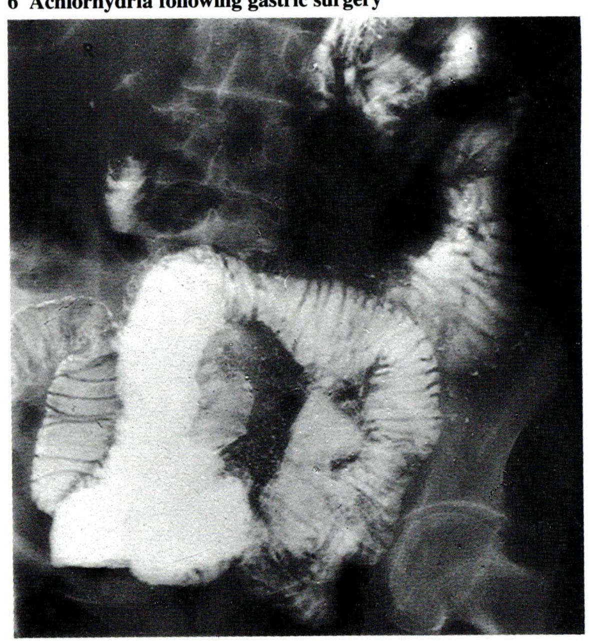

7 Cirrhosis and osteoporosis

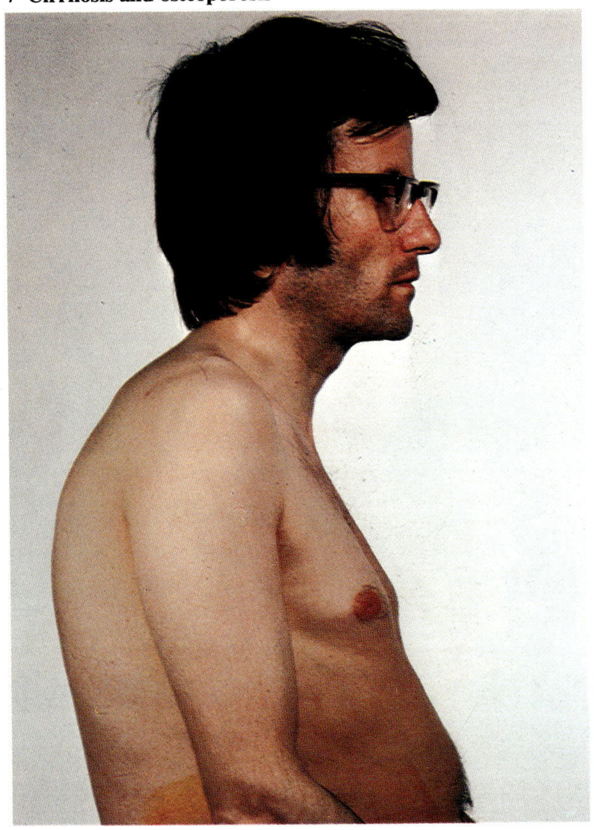

8 Steatorrhoea – pancreatic cysts

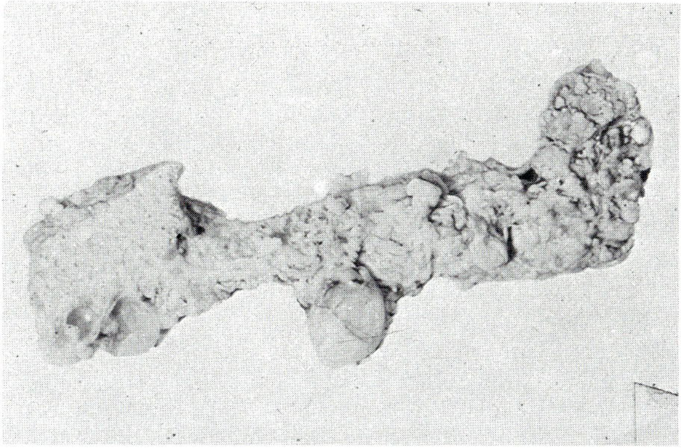

9 Coeliac disease

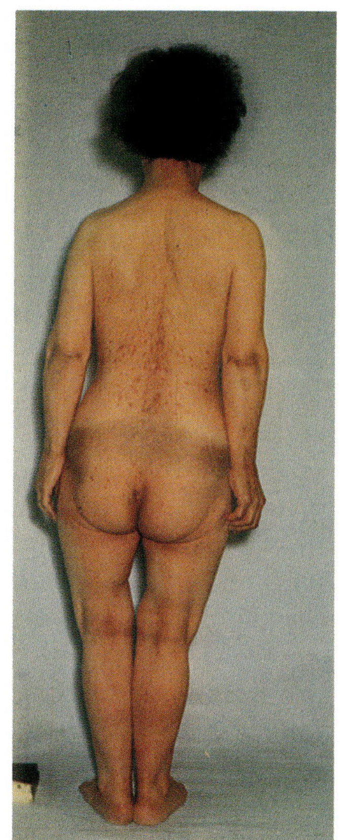

10 Sucrose barium meal

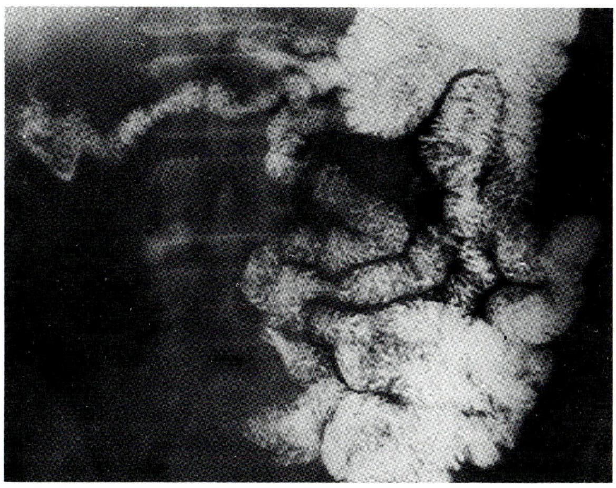

11 Lactose barium meal

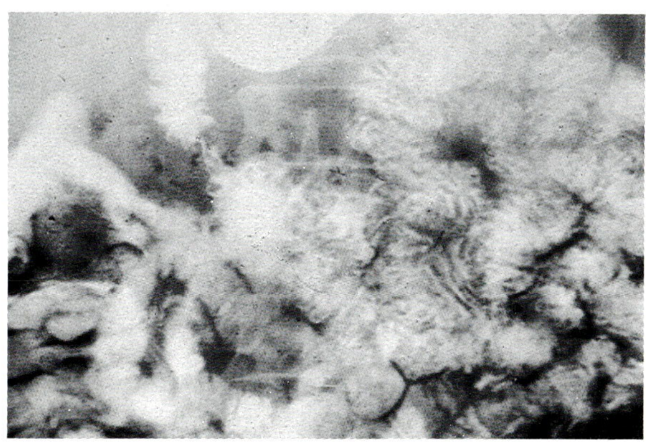

12 Calcium absorption and secretion

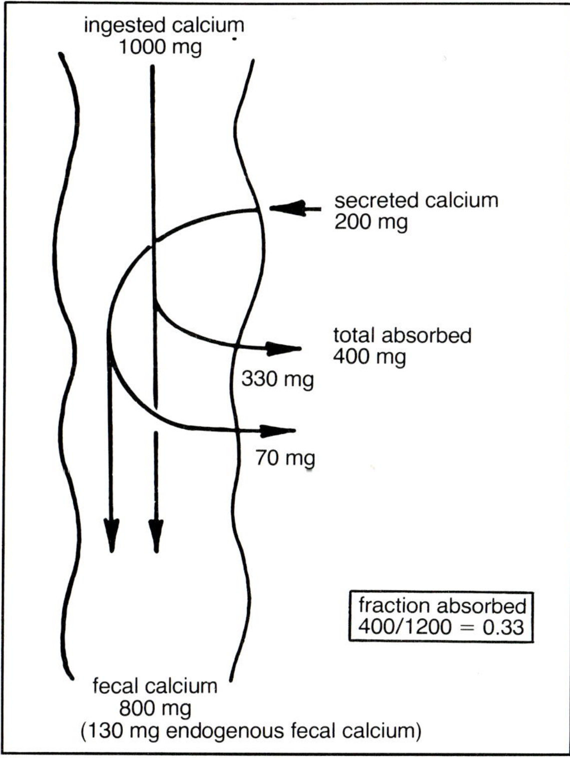

Luminal factors

- adequate calcium intake
- correct ratio of phosphate or phytate, an excess of either chelates calcium and prevents absorption
- sufficient acid to ionise calcium complexes, poor ionisation reduces absorption
- adequate lipolysis from pancreatic enzymes to prevent calcium loss from soaps in steatorrhoea causing a negative calcium balance
- no gross albumen loss into the lumen

Transport factors

Lumen is lined by a brush border containing the transport protein (CaBP) whose synthesis is dependent on the 1:25 OHCC concentration (**13**). Active transport of calcium is sensitive to a variety of drugs. Factors to be considered are:

- adequate luminal mucosa decreased in coeliac disease
- functional lymphatic system decreased in chylous ascites
- intact portal circulation decreased in Budd–Chiari syndrome and osteoporosis
- adequate circulating concentration of hormone (vitamin) D, 1:25 OH cholecalciferol
- absence of calcium transport inhibitors e.g. phenytoin sodium

13 Calcium transport factors

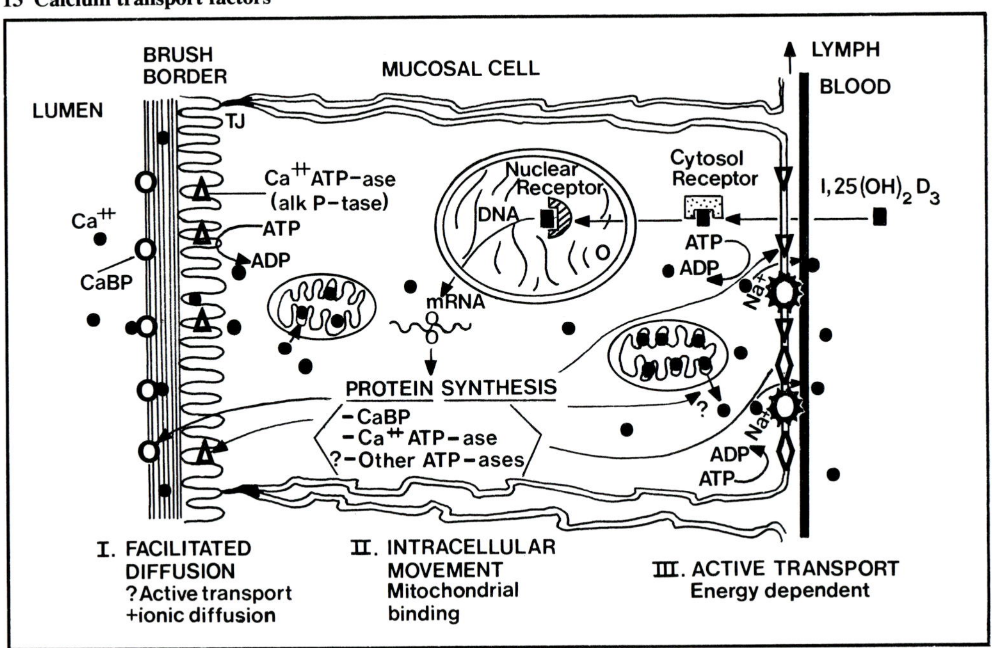

c. Survey and investigation for endocrine bone disease

A survey is then carried out to enquire about symptoms of endocrine dysfunction which disturbs bone synthesis.

1. Thyrotoxicosis, thyrotoxic facies and goitre (**14**)
2. Cushing's syndrome, purple striae and obesity with creases (**15**) suggesting vertebral collapse
3. Hyperparathyroidism, anxious slightly 'thyrotoxic look' of the hyperparathyroid patient (**16**)
4. Diabetes, (**17**) osteoporotic spine in 30 year old juvenile onset diabetic
5. Acromegaly, (**18**) showing the projecting jaw, (**19**) showing the spade-shaped hands against a normal hand

14 Thyrotoxicosis

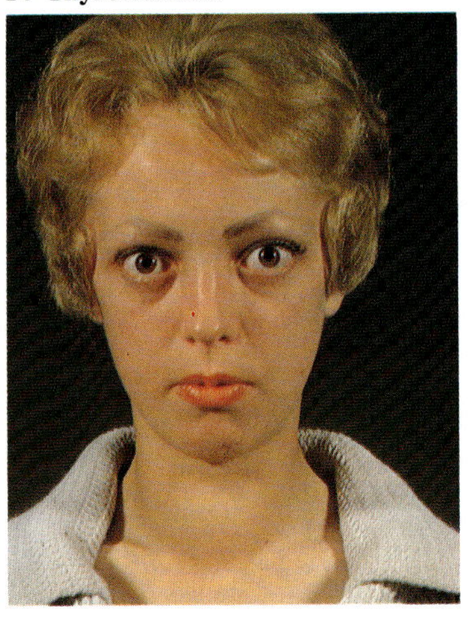

15 Cushing's syndrome

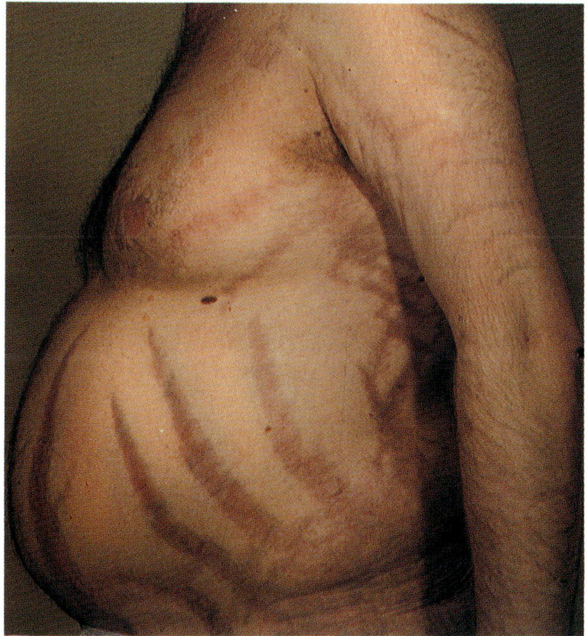

16 Hyperparathyroidism

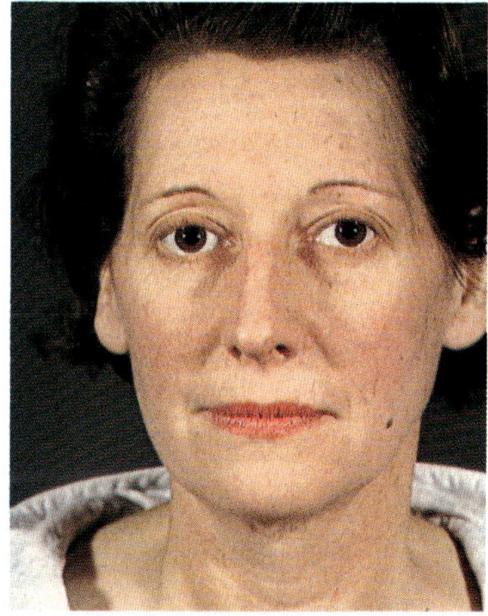

17 Diabetic osteoporosis

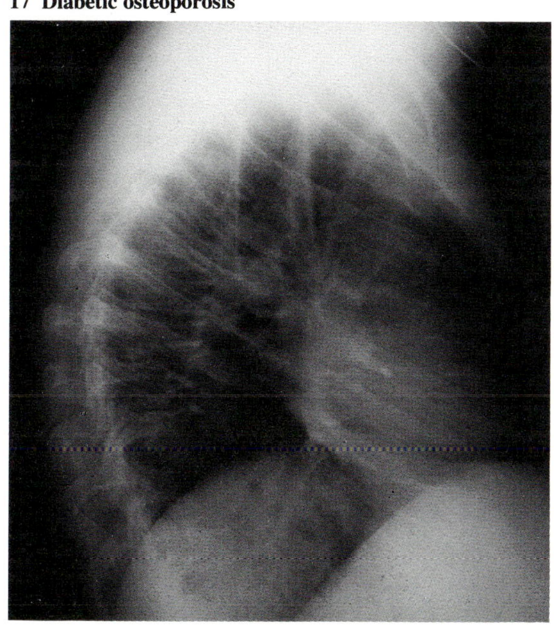

18 Acromegaly

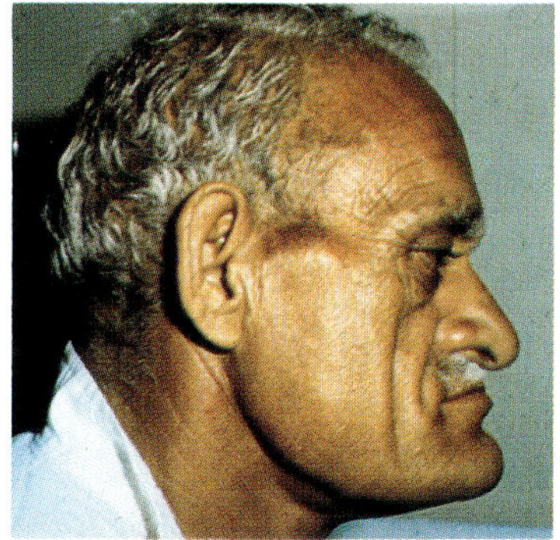

19 Acromegaly

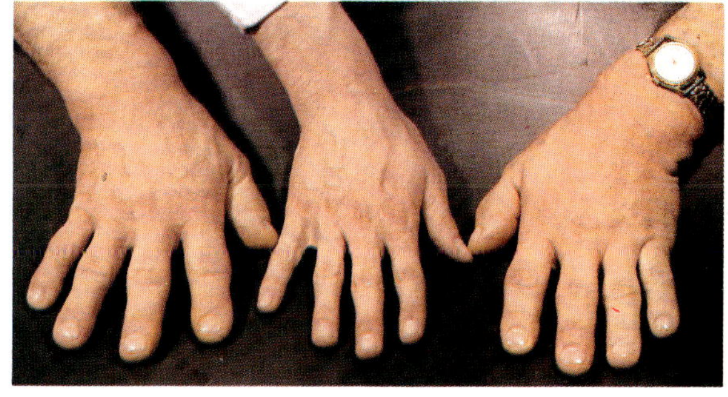

Suitable tests for each of the above:

i. Protein-bound iodine, triiodo thyronine, tetraiodo thyronine tests
ii. Fasting and nocturnal cortisols
iii. Estimation of immunoreactive parathyroid hormone, urinary cyclic adenosine monophosphate
iv. Glucose tolerance and immunoreactive insulin concentration tests
v. Estimation of immunoreactive growth hormone

These diseases may be masked as follows:

- by thoracic situated goitre or, in the elderly, a small nodule
- hypercorticosteroidism may be secondary to carcinoma producing adrenocorticotropic hormone
- hyperparathyroidism may not be detected by simple chemical tests because of vitamin D or Mg deficiency, and repletion with these may be necessary

Rarer endocrine mediated bone disease

1. Zollinger-Ellison syndrome
   - pleuriglandular syndrome
   - hypergastrinaemia
   - hypercalcaemia
2. Hypothyroidism – bone sclerosis
3. Pregnancy osteoporosis
4. Mastocytosis (**20**)
   - skin biopsy (**21** *Giemsa stain* × *160*) showing increased mast cells
   - bone biopsy (**22** *H&E* × *25*) showing mast cells and osteoporosis
5. Carcinoid, revealed by 5hydroxy indole acetic acid in urine

20 Mastocytosis in skin

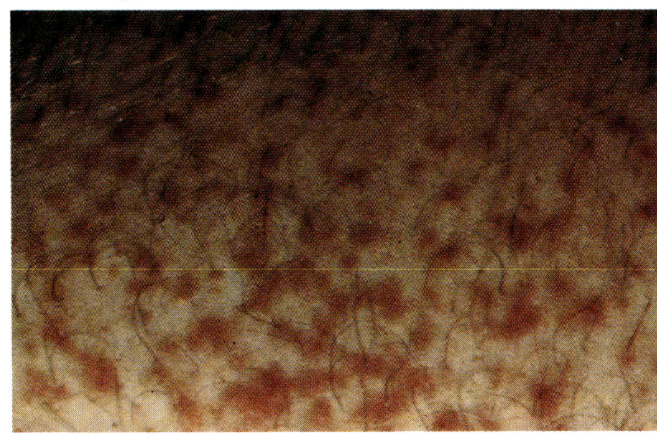

21 Mastocytosis in skin

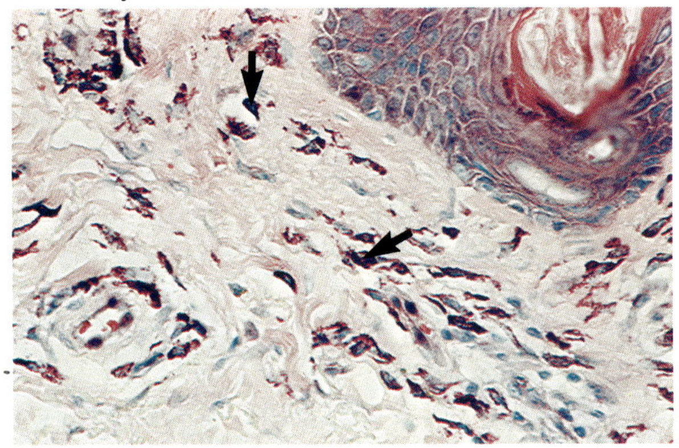

22 Osteoporosis in mastocytosis

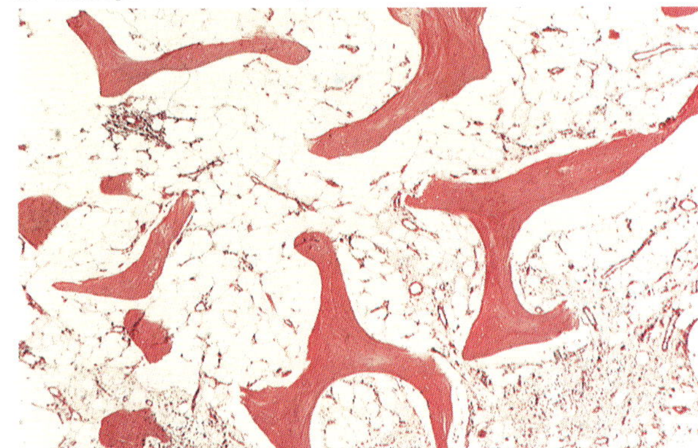

d. Survey and investigation for renal disease

A search should be made for symptoms and signs of renal disease which causes different types of bone disease. (Symptoms and signs of uraemia, **23**.)

1. Renal (glomerular) osteodystrophy

This can be caused by (**24**):
- loss of vitamin D binding protein in the nephrotic syndrome
- phosphate retention leading to 2^{0} hyperparathyroidism
- failure of hydroxylation of 25 OH cholecalciferol to 1:25 OHCC or 24:25 OHCC leading to osteomalacia
- loss of bone bicarbonate in chronic acidosis
- retention of toxic ions such as aluminium or fluoride leading to osteosclerosis and osteomalacia resistant to vitamin D
- effects of uraemic toxins on collagen formation leading to osteomalacia and osteoporosis

The main classes of this type of renal disease are nephritis, pyelonephritis, polycystic disease and chronic hypertension causing nephrosclerosis.

Glomerular failure is characterised by urea retention, phosphate retention (red eyes of uraemia, **25**), secondary hyperparathyroidism and bone disease (pseudoclubbing, **26**) and outer clavicular erosions (John Eager Howard sign, **27**.) This clinical triad is always indicative of advanced renal bone disease. Tumoural calcinosis occurs mainly in patients on regular dialysis therapy, (**28**) a deposit behind a patient's ear thought to be a tuberculous gland.

23 Uraemia – symptoms and signs

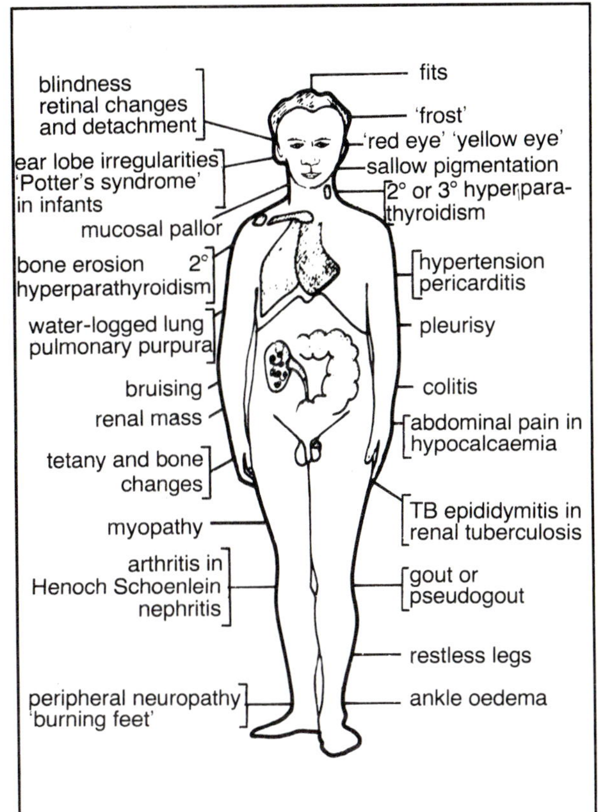

24 Renal bone disease – multiple factors

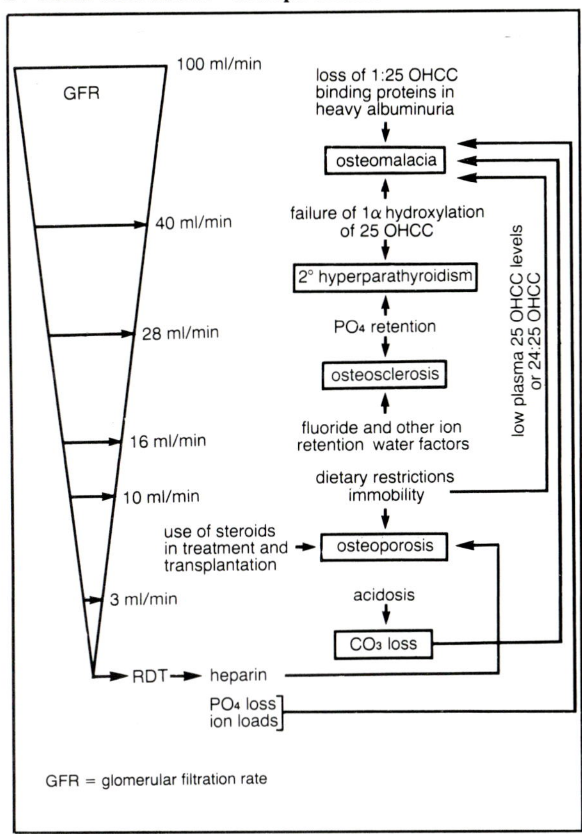

25 Red eye of uraemia

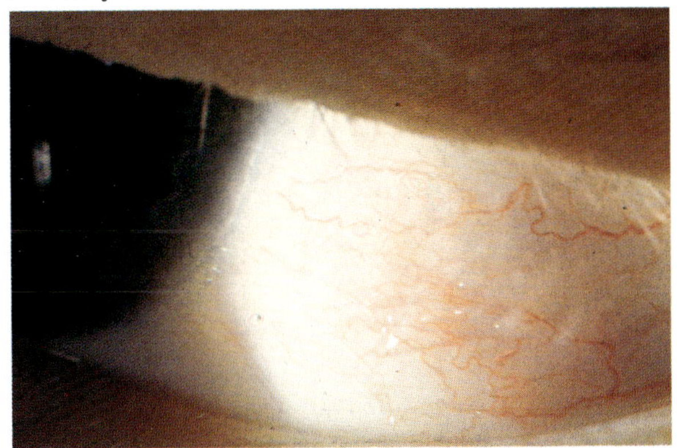

26 Pseudoclubbing

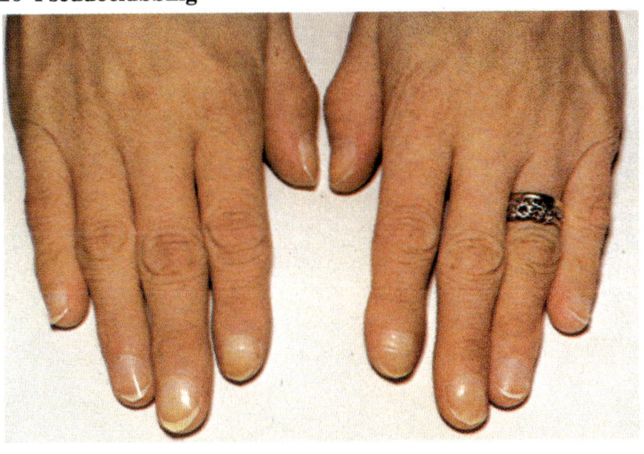

27 Clavicular erosions

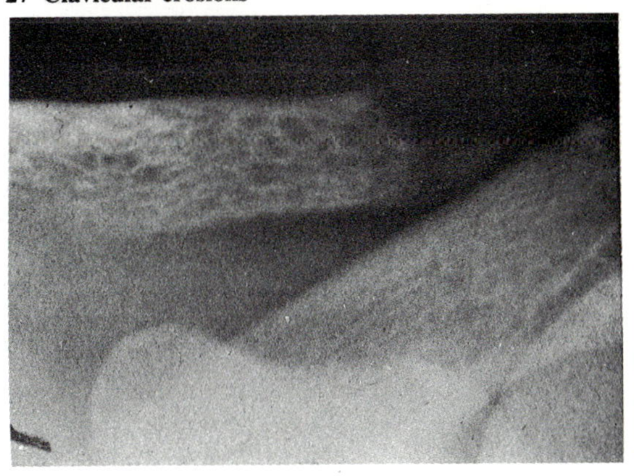

28 Tumoural calcinosis

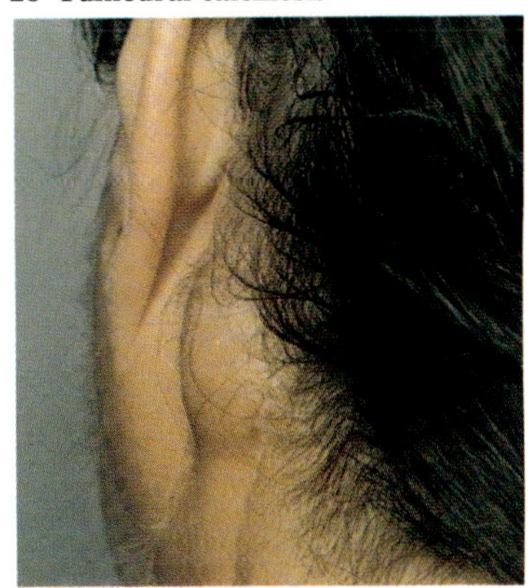

2. Renal tubular rickets (RTR) or osteomalacia

Urea retention is a late complication of renal tubular rickets. Many of the tubular defects exist early in skeletal development and lead to severe stunting in growth and abnormal upper segment/lower segment ratios. This 18 year old boy is 1.52 m tall (**29**). Many are also associated with failure of tubular phosphate transport possibly linked with failure of 1α hydroxylation of vitamin D and are called vitamin D resistant rickets or malacia.

29 Renal tubular rickets

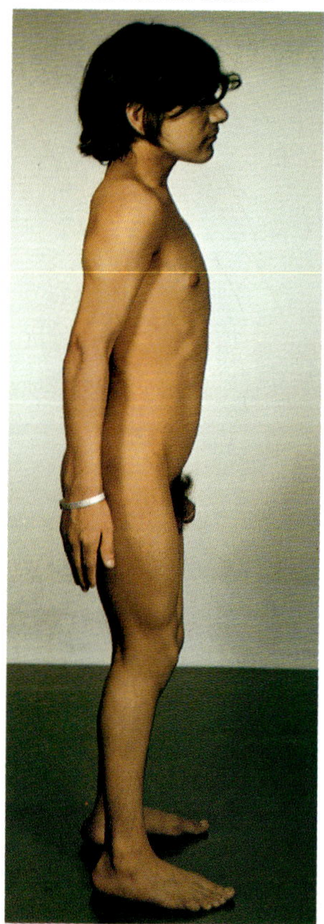

Types of renal tubular rickets include:

i. Vitamin D resistant RTR (phosphate losing) in a 6 year old girl (**30**) showing bone deformity
   - presenting as an infant sex linked or steroid sensitive syndrome
   - adult presenting (some with hyperglycaemia)
   - associated with neurofibromatosis (**31**)

ii. Fanconi's syndrome, aminoaciduria and phosphaturia, swollen wrists (**32**)

iii. Lowe's syndrome, rickets with mental retardation and glaucoma (**33**)

iv. Butler Albright syndrome
   - aminoaciduria
   - phosphaturia and renal tubular acidosis (RTA)

v. Albright's polyostotic fibrous dysplasia with osteomalacia
   - cystic bony changes
   - skin pigmentation (Coast of Maine) (**34**)
   - precocious puberty
   - occasional hypophosphataemia

vi. Acquired Fanconi-like syndromes
   - cystinosis
   - myeloma
   - heavy metal tubular toxins (copper and lead)
   - severe vitamin D deficiency

30 Renal tubular rickets – phosphate losing

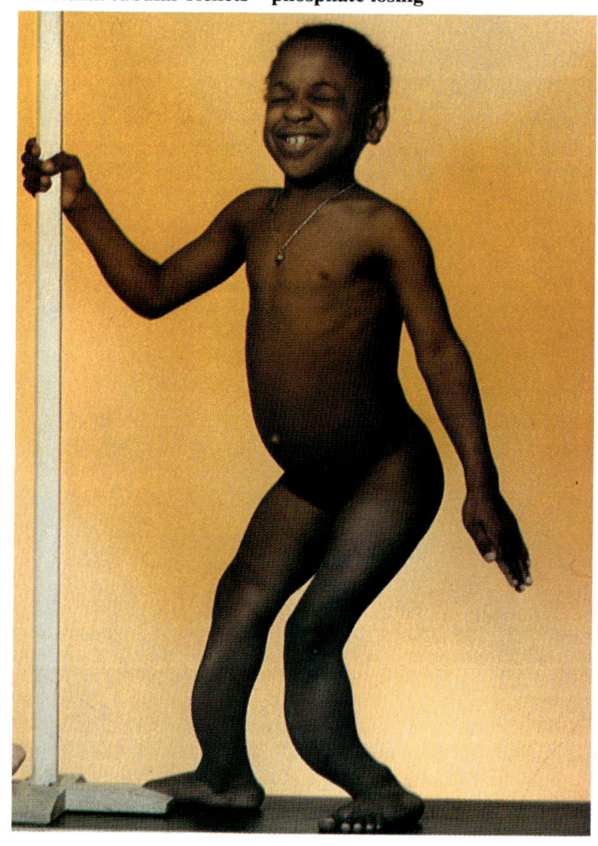

31 **Neurofibromatosis**

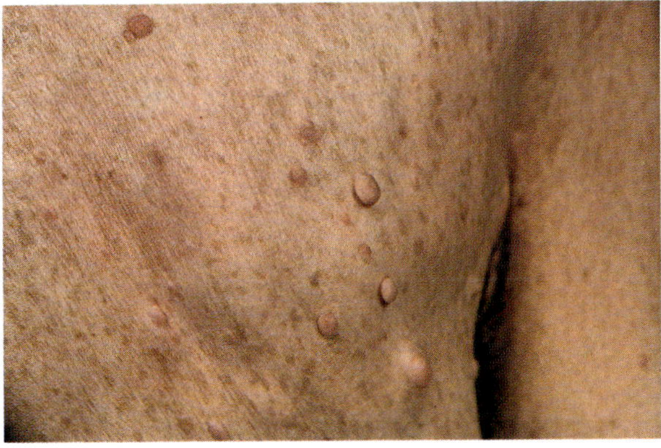

32 **Fanconi's syndrome**

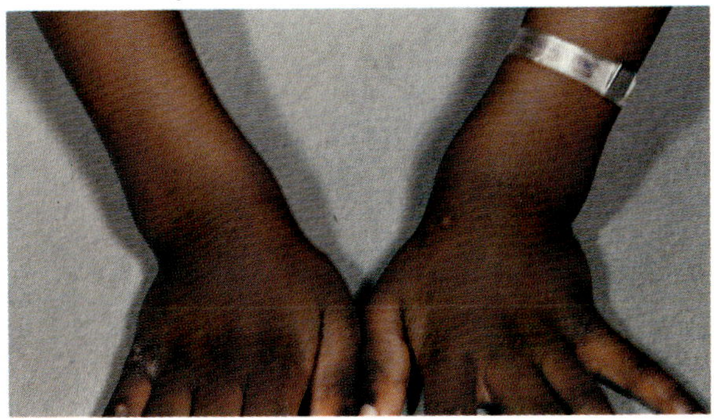

33 **Lowe's syndrome**

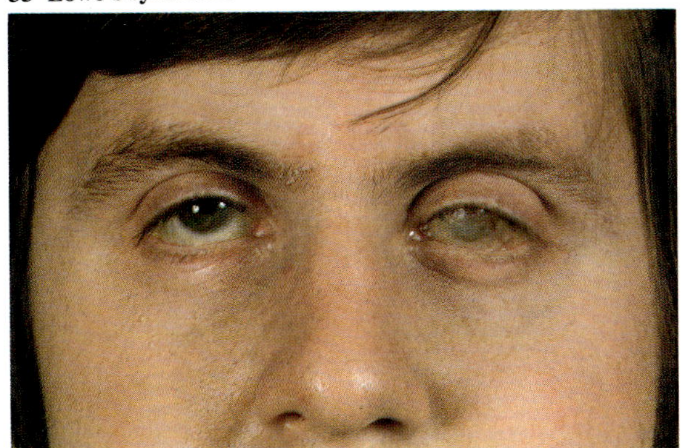

34 **Coast of Maine skin pigmentation**

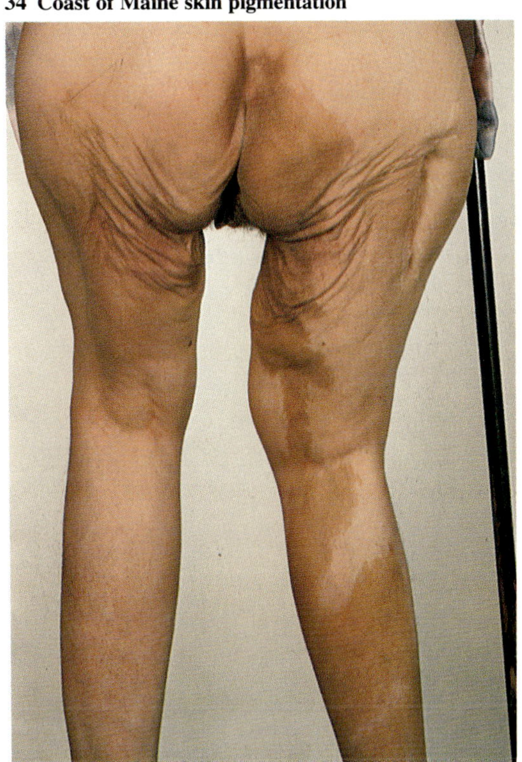

e. Bone signs in systemic disease

1. Osteomyelitis
   - from the umbilicus in the new born
   - from septic foci such as pneumonia, subacute bilateral endocarditis
   - from the gut e.g. Salmonella in sickle-cell disease
   - from tuberculosis elsewhere in the body
   - from syphilis or yaws infection
2. Osteonecrosis
   - secondary to multiple system disease such as disseminated lupus erythematosis
   - secondary to steroid administration following transplantation, (**35**) scan from a transplanted patient with early osteonecrosis of the femoral head which picks up isotope more avidly than the surrounding pelvic bones
   - due to compressed air disease

35 **Osteonecrosis of femoral head**

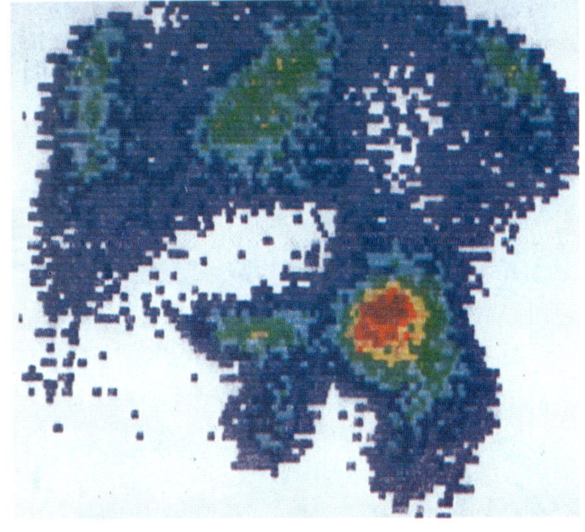

f. Symptoms of malignant disease

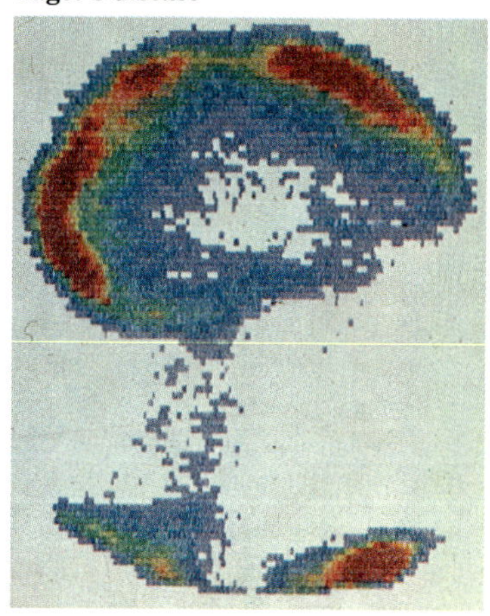

36 Bone scan – sarcoma of skull in Paget's disease

A search should be made for symptoms associated with the commoner malignant diseases in the appropriate age range.

1. Chest symptoms or operations
2. Breast symptoms, signs or operations
3. Symptoms suggestive of stomach neoplasm
4. Urological symptoms suggestive of carcinoma of the prostate
5. A change in bowel habit suggestive of malignant disease of the colon
6. Loss of weight, back pain suggestive of carcinoma of the pancreas
7. Fever, itching, alcohol intolerance suggestive of lymphoma
8. Skin markers of malignancy

Investigations include:
- calcium, phosphate, acid and alkaline phosphatases (see table below)
- urinary OH proline excretion
- bone scan (**36**)
- exfoliative cytology
- bone biopsy of hot spots in scan

Typical blood and urine findings

Type of tumour	Ca.	PO4	Acid PO4ase	Alk/ PO4ase	Urinary OH proline	Blood film
Breast	N or ↑	N	N	↑	↑	N or LE
Bronchus	N or ↑	N or ↓	N or ↑	↑	↑	N or LE
Prostate	N	N	↑	N or ↑	↑	N
Stomach	N or ↑	N	N	↑	↑	N or LE
Thyroid	N	N	N	↑	N or ↑	N
Myeloma	N or ↑	N or ↓	N	N	N	Rouleaux +++
Leukaemia	N or ↑	N	N	N	N or ↑	WBC ↑

N normal. ↑ raised. ↓ lowered. LE leucoerythroblastic.
WBC white blood cell count.

g. Bone disease as an occupational hazard

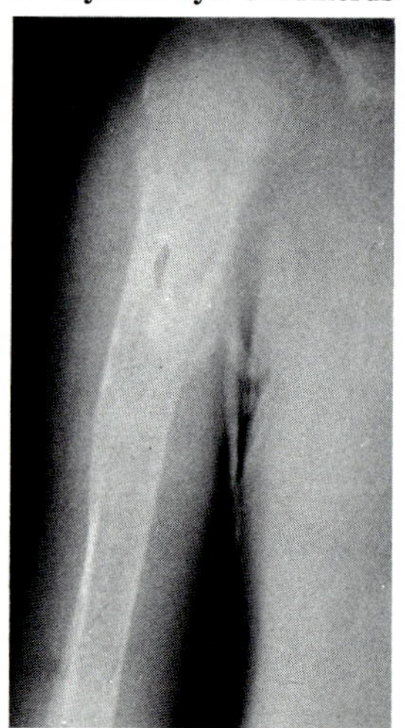

37 Hydatid cyst in humerus

1. Footballers – trauma, often around the knee joint
2. Compressed air divers – bone necrosis in femora
3. Meat porters – hydatid (**37**) involving viscera and bone
4. Radiation workers – bone lesions from exposure to the hands
5. Aluminium smelters – fluorosis from inhaled aluminium and fluoride leads to bone sclerosis

h. Family history of bone or connective tissue disease

1. Diseases affecting collagen synthesis. Osteogenesis imperfecta congenita and osteogenesis imperfecta tarda, the first, more severe type affecting a young child causing gross deformity. Compare normal sclerae with **55**
2. Diseases affecting mucopolysaccharide synthesis (see table on page 84)
3. Diseases affecting elastic tissue and, indirectly, bone growth e.g. Marfan's syndrome
4. Diseases of bone growth and maturation – diaphyseal dysplasia, epiphyseal dysplasia, (**38**) a severely afflicted child with bossing of the skull, faintly blue sclerae and chest and limb deformities

38 Epiphyseal dysplasia

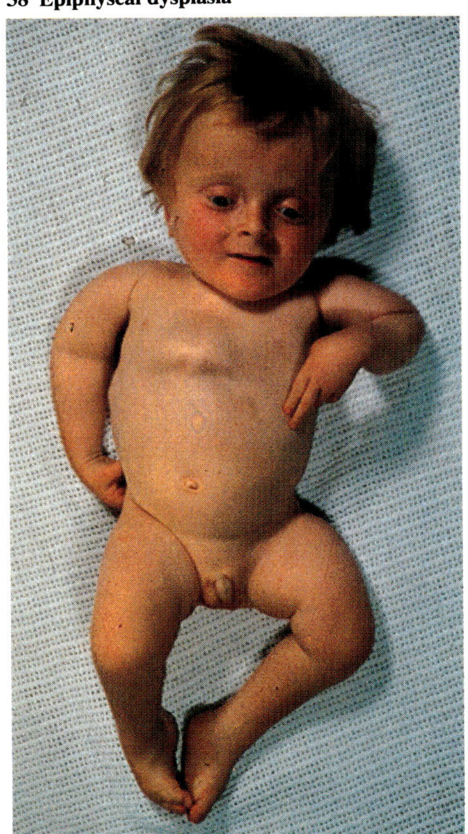

i. Symptomatic pathological fracture

A pathological fracture is one that occurs, mostly in response to trivial trauma, through a bone weakened by some underlying disease. The disease may be a generalised one such as osteoporosis, or a localised one such as a carcinoma metastasis. A pathological fracture of the upper humerus due to osteosarcoma, a primary neoplasm of bone (**39**). Different causes of pathological fracture predominate at different ages, see table below.

39 Fracture due to osteosarcoma

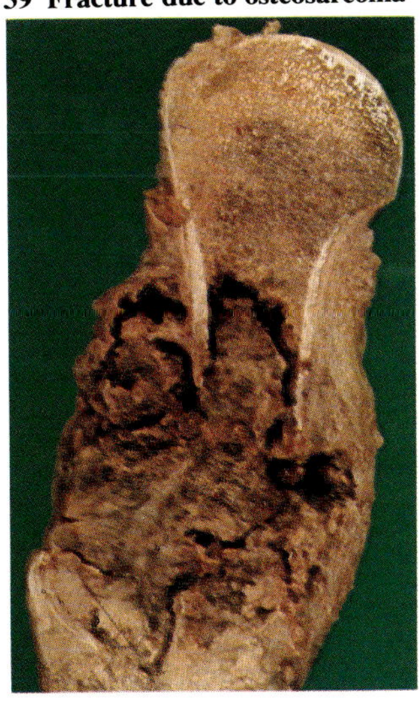

Pathological fracture – causes

Infancy	Childhood	Adult life
osteogenesis imperfecta	rickets	osteoporosis
scurvy	osteomyelitis	osteomalacia
congenital rickets	fibrous defects	Paget's disease
metaphyseal fibrous defect	Gaucher's disease	metastases to bone
osteopetrosis	osteosarcoma	primary bone neoplasm
	eosinophilic granuloma	bone cysts
	non-ossifying fibroma	aseptic bone necrosis
	simple bone cyst	ionising radiation
		hyperparathyroidism
		fibrous defects
		massive bone osteolysis

2. Examination of the patient

a. General examination

For many patients a full system examination will have been made and no account will be given of these procedures, but particular attention should be given to the examination of abnormalities of soft tissues and the bones beneath.

The estimation of height and span is important. Leonardo da Vinci's diagram (**40**) represents the relationship of span to height and the consequent symmetry.

This leads to a clinical measurement of the span from head to hand, of the upper segment of height from crown to pubis and of the lower segment of height from pubis to heel (**41**). Bone diseases which cause a severe retardation in growth affect height more than span.

Where the disease has occurred during adolescence and has affected the weight-bearing bones, the upper segment/lower segment ratio may alter causing an apparent shortening of the lower segment. The hands appear to reach the knees in this boy with renal tubular rickets (**42**).

40 Bodily symmetry

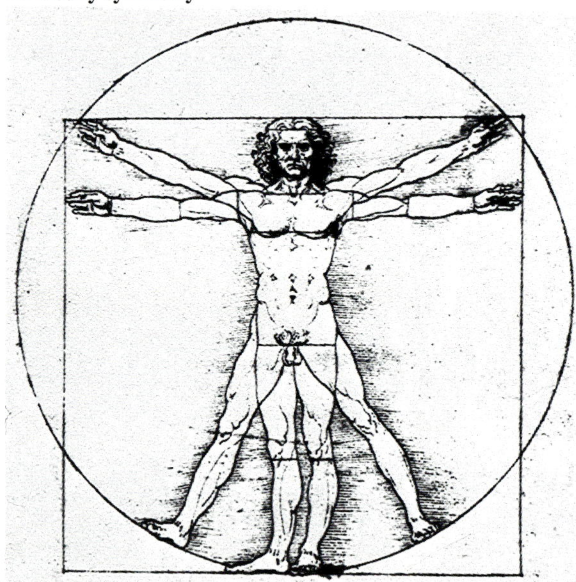

41 Measurement of lower segment length

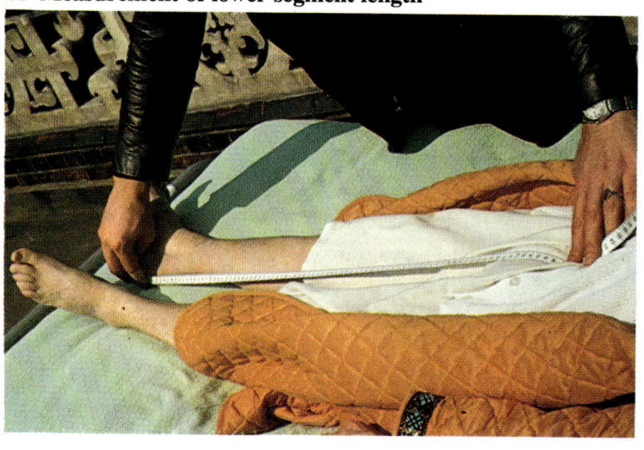

42 Renal tubular rickets – shortening of lower segment

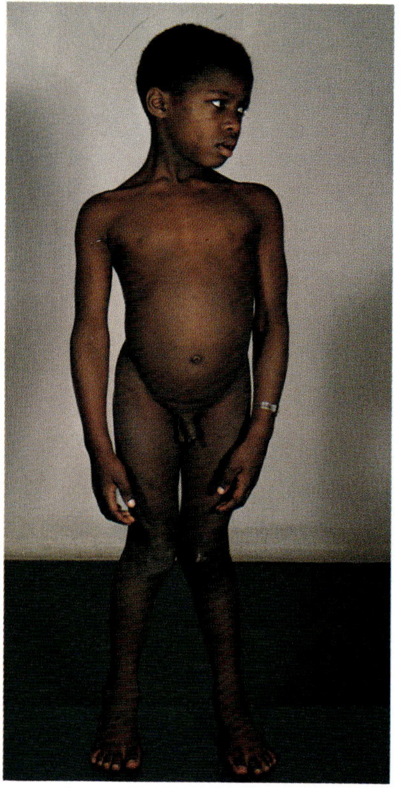

Bone disease acquired later in life can also give rise to a similar shrinking of the upper segment causing the hands to reach the knees (**43**).

When carried out serially these measurements are useful in detecting changes in deformity and vertebral collapse. Progressive loss of height indicates progressive loss of vertebral height.

Alterations in the degree of deformity may encourage therapy to be continued. The improvement in knock knees over a period of 2 years in a child with rickets is shown in **44**.

Examination of the limbs may reveal the characteristic bowing of the tibiae seen in Paget's disease (**45**) or syphilis, or a massive cystic swelling from rheumatoid arthritis (**46**).

43 Osteoporosis – shortening of upper segment

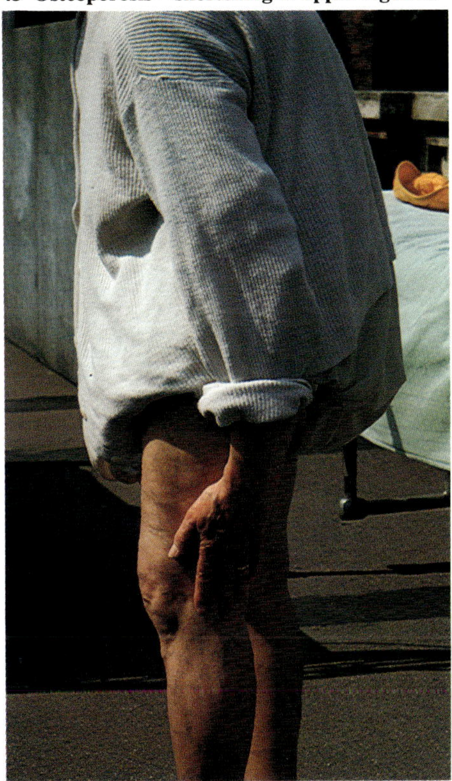

45 Paget's disease – bowing of tibiae

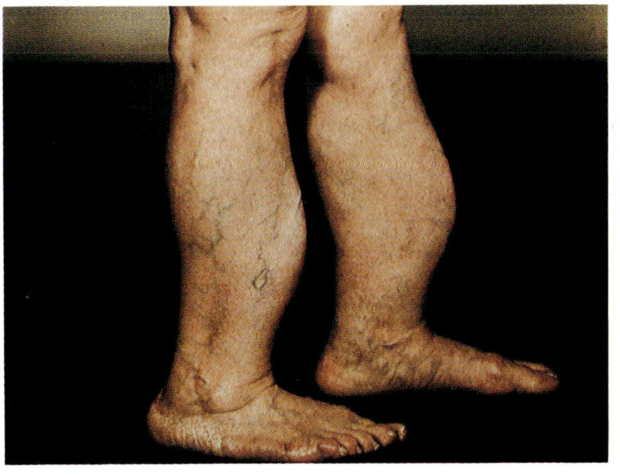

44 Phosphate losing rickets – knock knees

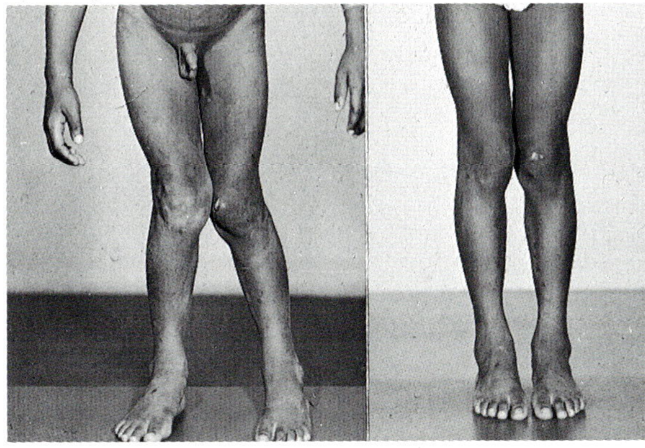

46 Rheumatoid cystic swelling

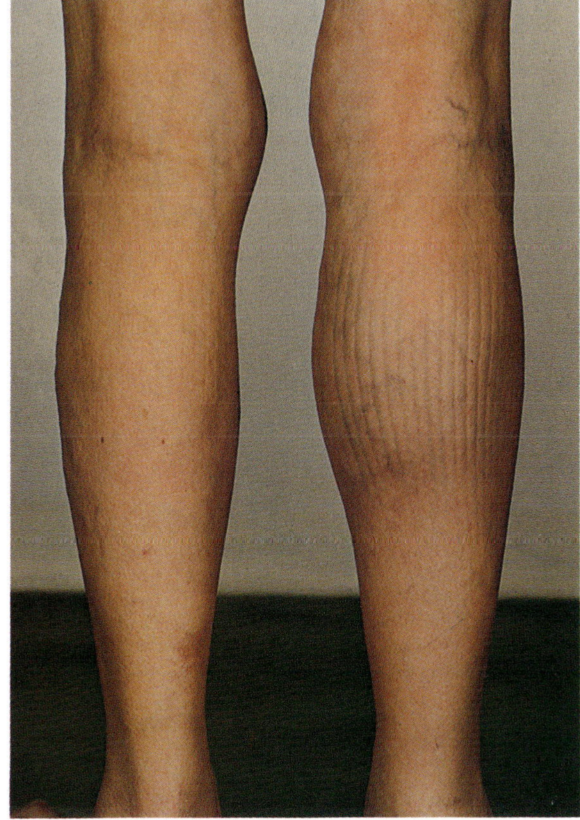

Nail, skin and hair changes are common in bone disease. Nail abnormalities with absent patellae are linked to renal glomerular defects, the nail-patella syndrome (**47**). Brittle nails with gross ridging are seen in advanced osteoporosis (**48**), thin fragile ulcerating skin in malabsorption and osteomalacia (**49**) and chronic moniliasis in hypoparathyroidism (**50**).

Thin fragile skin with senile purpura and prominent tendons are associated with osteoporosis with or without steroid treatment for rheumatoid arthritis, McConkey's sign (**51**).

Neurofibromatosis can be associated with osteomalacia (**52**).

Haemangiomas of the gut can be associated with osteomas of bone, Gardner's syndrome.

Occasionally the hair becomes thin and brittle (**53**).

47 Renal glomerular defect – nail-patella syndrome

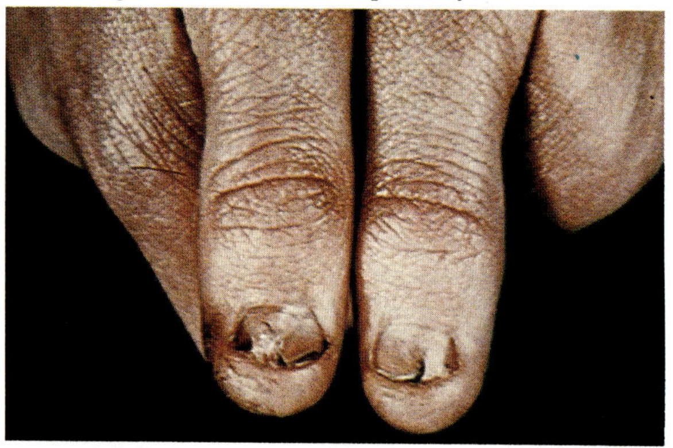

48 Osteoporosis – ridged nails

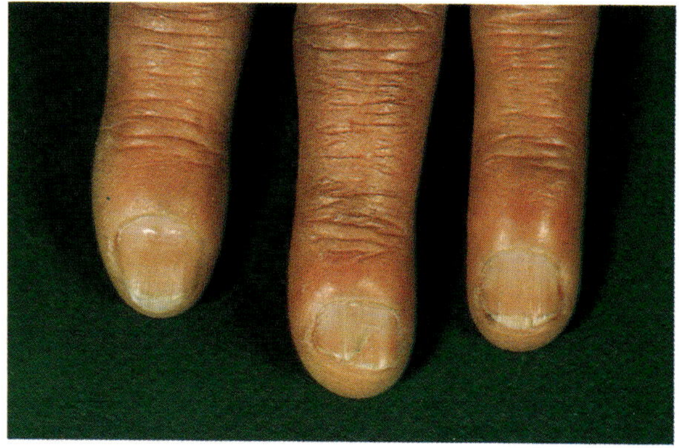

49 Osteomalacia – fragile ulcerating skin

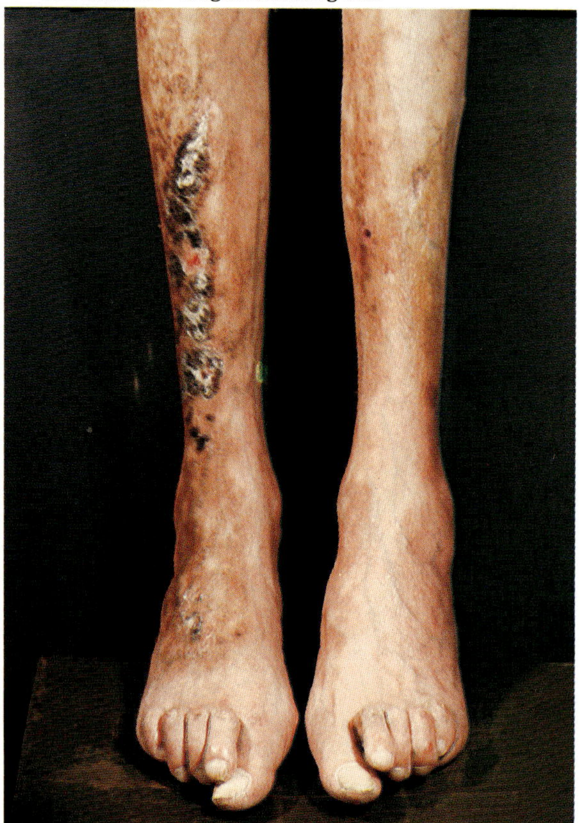

50 Hypoparathyroidism – chronic moniliasis

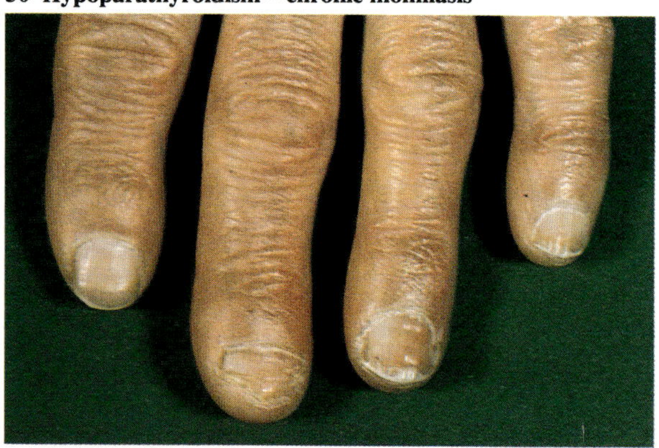

51 Osteoporosis – thin fragile skin

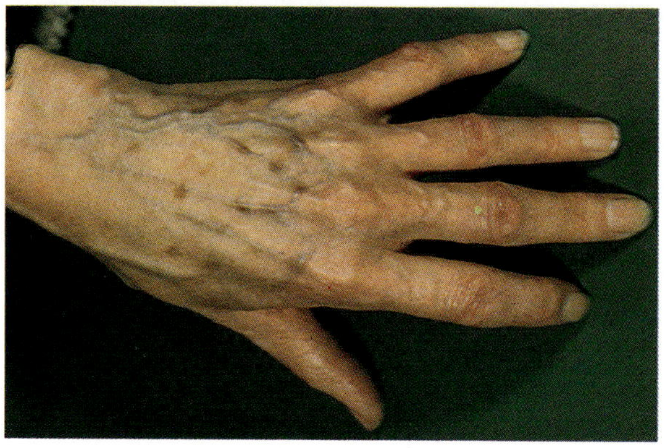

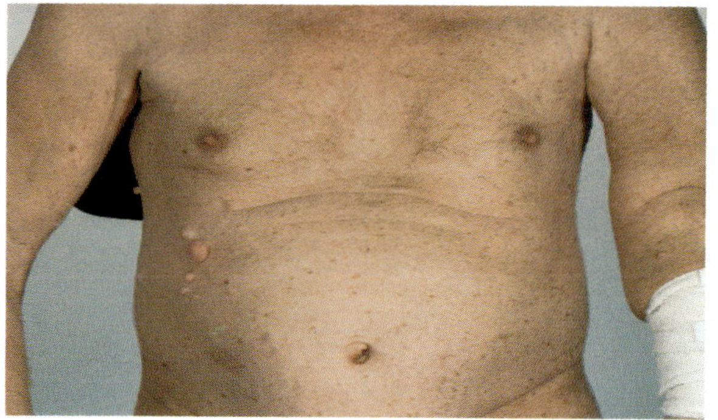

52 Neurofibromatosis

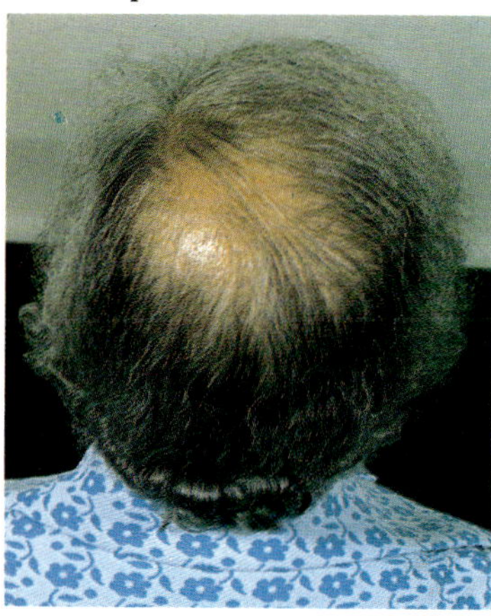

53 Osteoporosis – brittle hair

Examination of the eyes may reveal:
- band keratopathy of hypercalcaemia (**54**)
- 'red eyes' of uraemia due to hyperphosphataemia (see **25**)
- grey-blue sclerae of osteogenesis imperfecta (**55**)
- evidence of systemic disease occasionally affecting bone such as sarcoidosis, a sarcoid follicle seen in the iris (**56**)
- characteristic lens opacities with some varieties of mucopolysaccharidosis and hydrocephalus (**57**)
- angioid streaks in the retina of some patients with Paget's disease

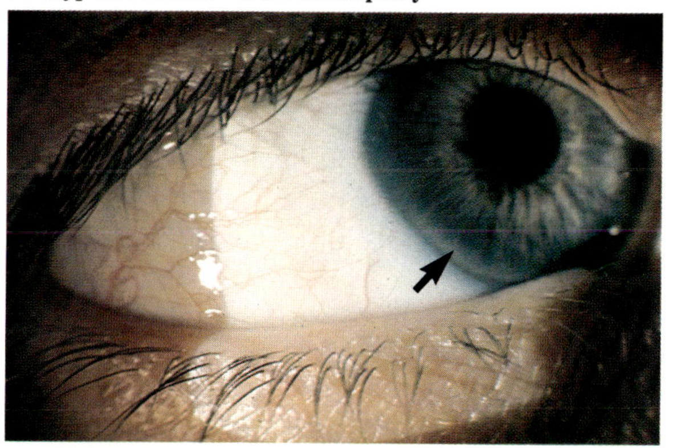

54 Hypercalcaemia – band keratopathy

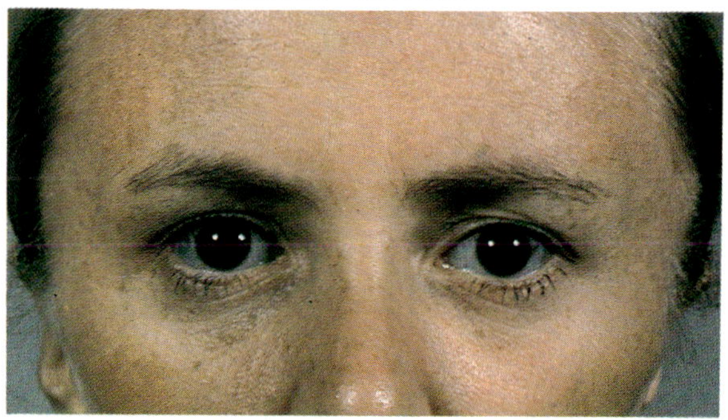

55 Osteogenesis imperfecta – blue sclerae

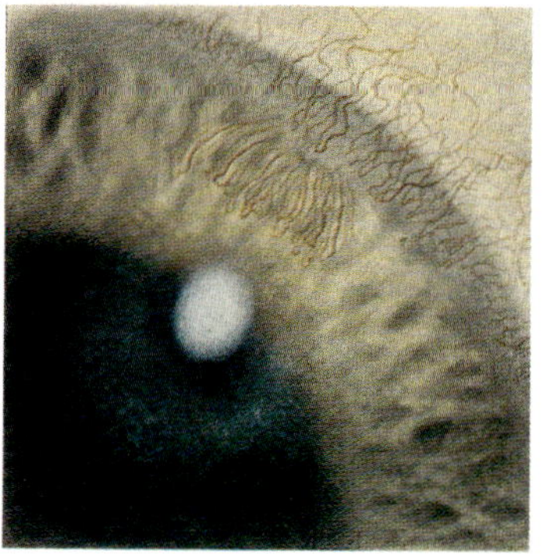

56 Sarcoidosis of iris

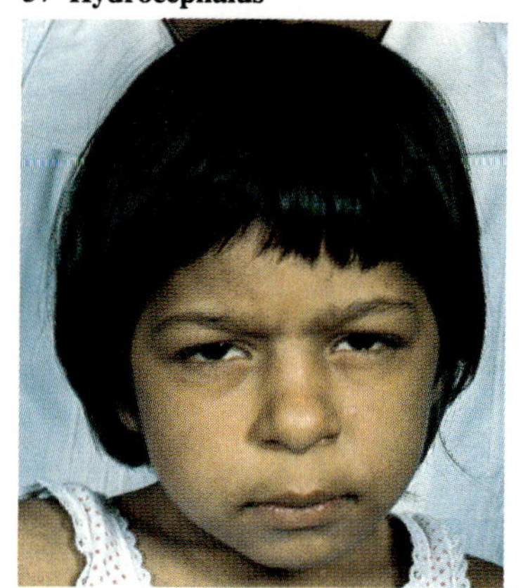

57 Hydrocephalus

Finally, when taking the blood pressure the cuff can be left on to produce spasm of the fingers, 'main d'accoucheur', of hypocalcaemic tetany (**58**). A brisk jerk with deviation of the mouth is known as 'Chvostek's masseter sign' of hypocalcaemia.

Gross proximal myopathy can accompany osteomalacia (**59**).

Occasionally a bony tumour can be seen. A patient with a 'brown tumour' secondary to hyperparathyroidism (**60**).

58 Hypocalcaemic tetany – 'main d'accoucheur'

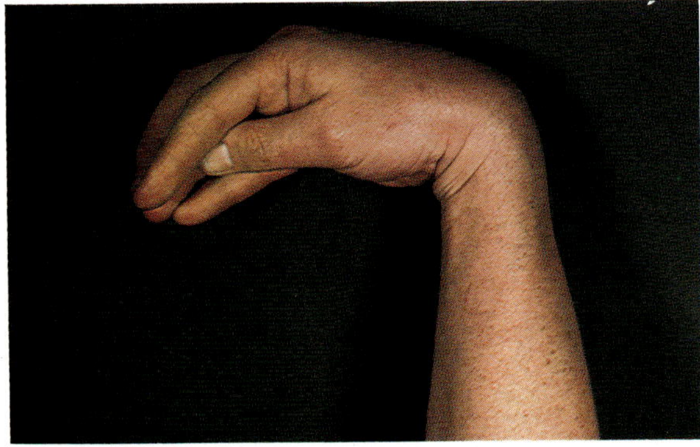

60 Brown tumour in lower jaw

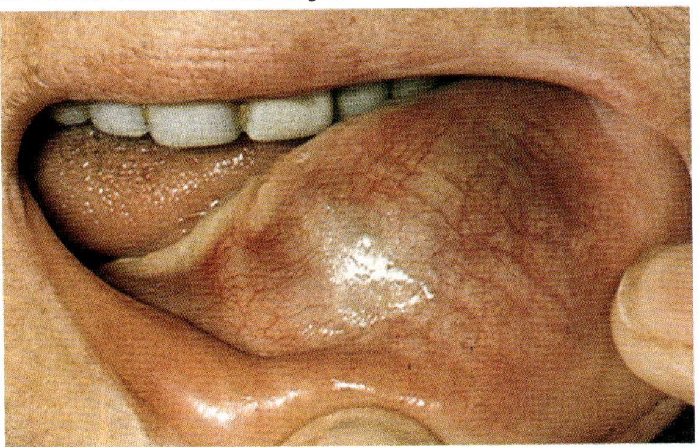

59 Renal osteomalacia – gross myopathy

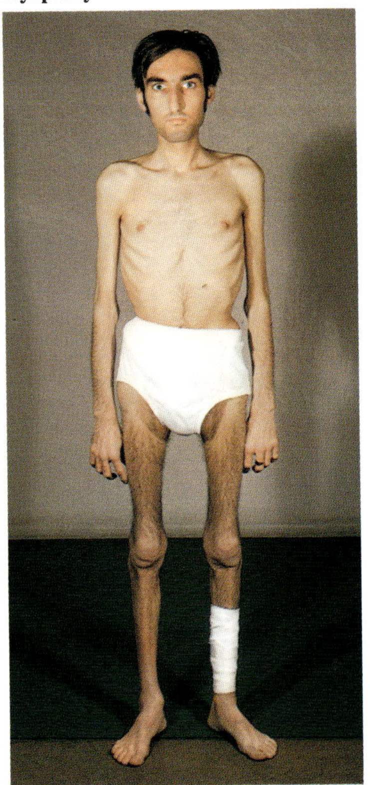

b. Initial investigations

It is difficult to determine priorities in the investigation of a patient presenting with bone symptoms but radiology, haematology and biochemistry are mandatory. Subsequent investigations are chosen according to the initial diagnosis and include bone scans, histology and density measurements.

1. Radiology

Although the main effort will be directed to the bone or bones giving rise to symptoms, it is useful to include views of:

- the chest, for changes in ribs, clavicles and scapulae. Diffuse sclerosis in all bones due to carcinoma of breast (**61**)
- the hands, metacarpal cortical thickness changes can be measured (**62**). Changes following treatment for Paget's disease are shown in **63**
- the skull, for changes and erosions of metabolic and haematological disease, myeloma of skull (**64**)
- the alveolar bone, particularly for hyperparathyroidism, (**65**, **66**) showing resorption of the dense line surrounding the teeth. In Paget's disease there is hypercementosis (**67**)
- the upper parts of the femora, for pseudofractures (**68**)

61 Diffuse sclerosis due to carcinoma of breast

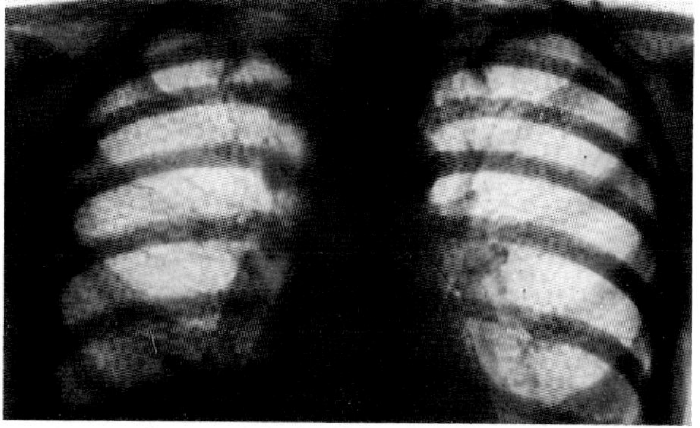

62 Metacarpal cortical thickness changes

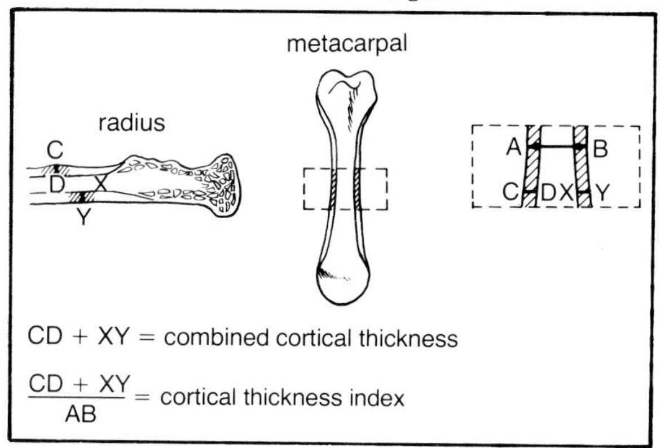

63 Cortical thickness changes following treatment for Paget's disease

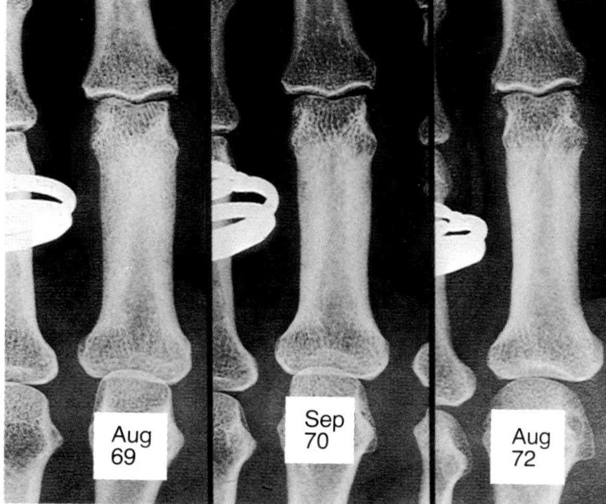

64 Myeloma of skull

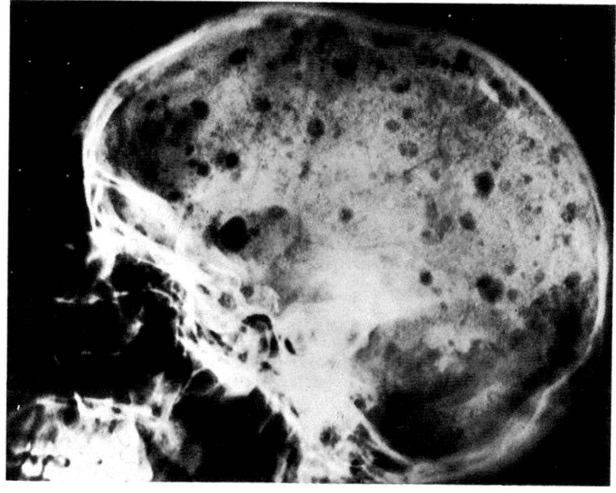

65 Secondary hyperparathyroidism – no lamina densa

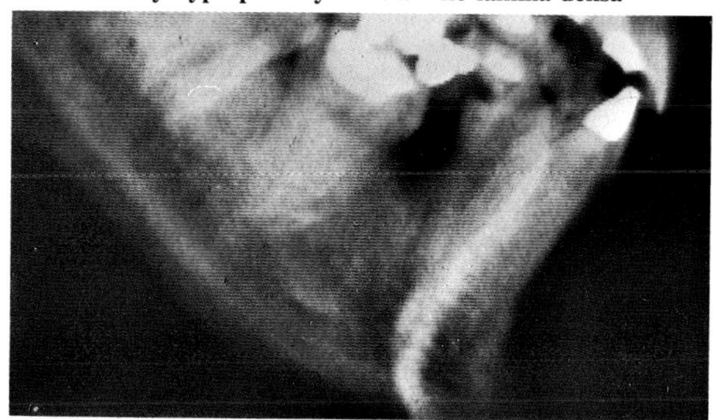

66 Primary hyperparathyroidism – missing laminae

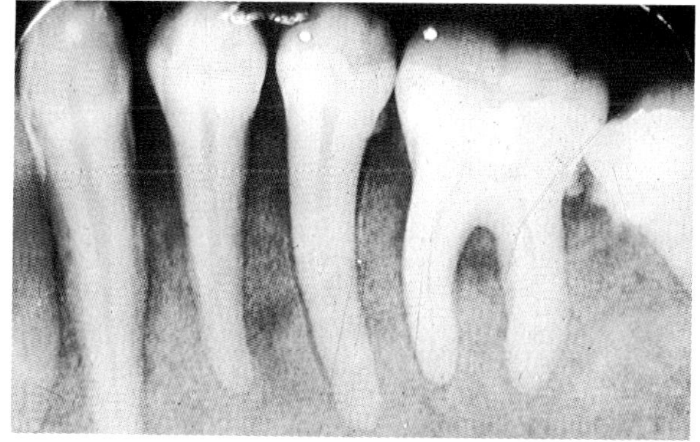

67 Paget's disease – hypercementosis around molar tooth

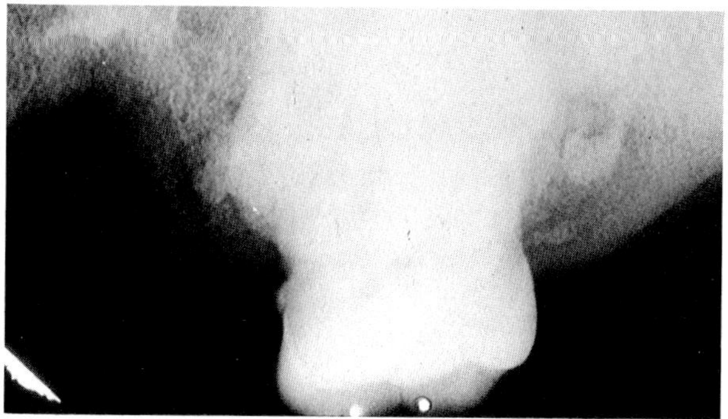

68 Multiple pseudofractures in osteomalacia

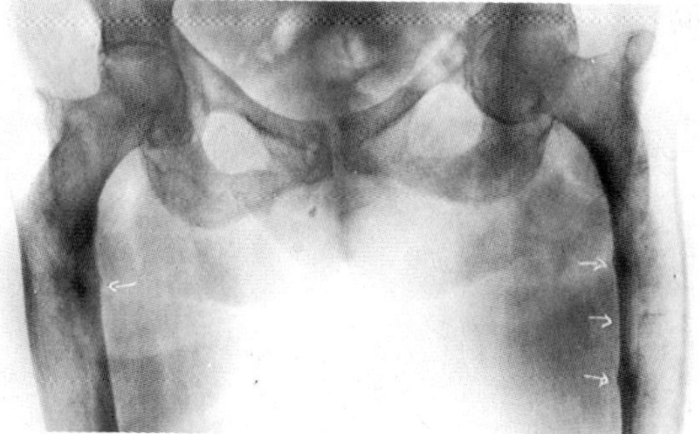

2. Haematological investigations

These are limited but include:

- erythrocyte sedimentation rate, raised in immunological disease, myeloma and malignancy
- haemoglobin, especially for anaemia, evidence of malabsorption, blood loss, uraemia, sickle cell disease
- white cell count for evidence of osteomyelitis, leukaemia or leucoerythroblastic anaemia due to metastases
- blood film, for sickle cells (**69**), Burr cells

69 Blood film – sickle cells

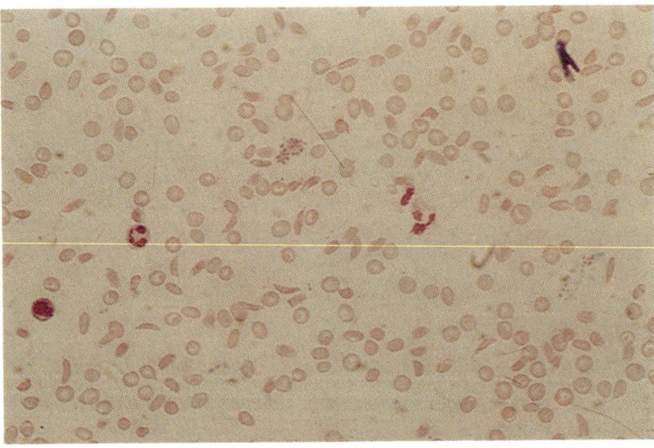

3. Biochemical investigations

(Optional investigations are in brackets)

- calcium phosphate, alkaline phosphatase (fractionated) (**70**)
- albumen, total proteins, (protein electrophoresis) and immunoglobulins
- 24 hour urine for calcium phosphate, creatinine, (hydroxyproline)
- aliquot of urine for amino acids, (mucopolysaccharide screen)
- (renal acidification tests where required)

70 Plasma chemistry in bone disease

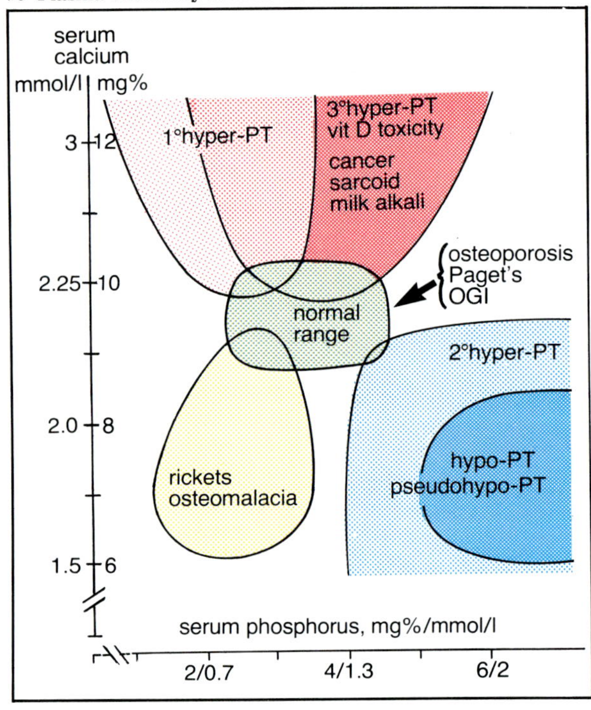

4. Tomography and arteriography

The differential diagnosis of bone tumours is greatly helped by tomography and arteriography.

5. Multitone imaging

Various isotopes are used according to the information required and how often the scan is to be repeated.

- isotopes Sr^{85} used rarely now, usually to follow turnover in a tumour deposit. Pelvis and hip with metastases (**71**)

F^{18} taken up by soft tissue tumours and bone, of use in following sarcoma metastases
Tnm^{99} DPTA routine wholebody scans for metabolic disease and metastases, normal (**72**), secondary deposits (**73**)

71 Sr^{85} scan – metastases in pelvis and hip

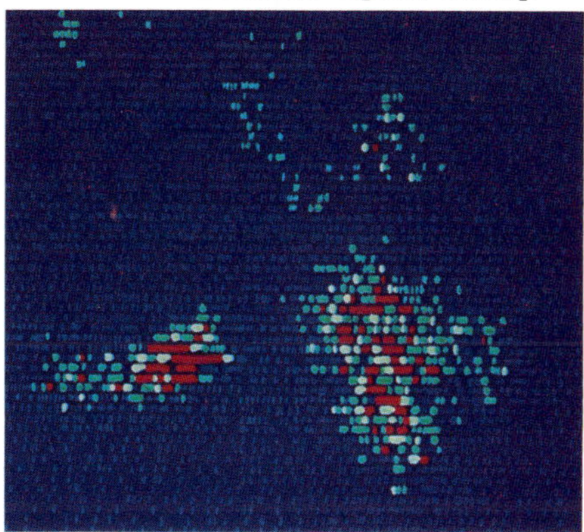

72 Tnm^{99} scan – normal

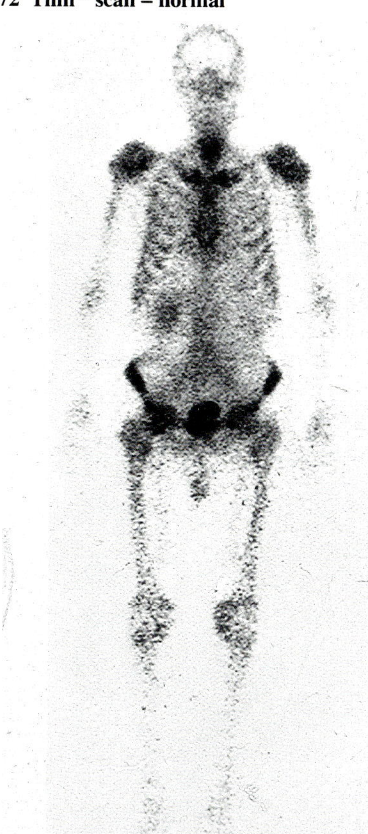

73 Tnm^{99} DPTA scan – deposits

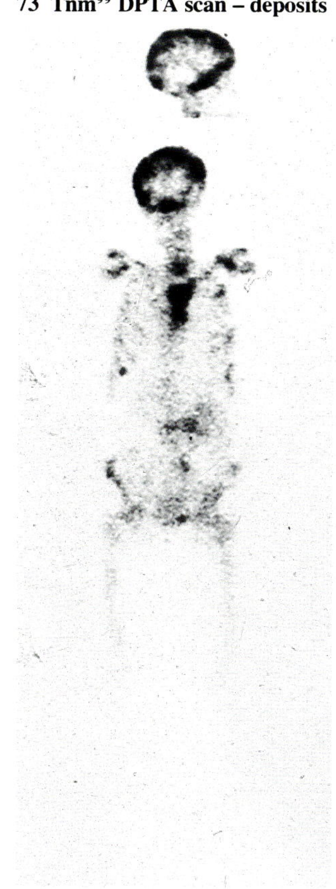

- indication for use of scans:
  - to detect the extent of skeletal involvement in metabolic bone disease e.g. renal osteodystrophy
  - to monitor the results of therapy on widespread disease e.g. Paget's disease
  - to detect the presence and extent of primary and secondary tumours of bone
  - to follow the effects of cytotoxic therapy and radiotherapy on such tumour deposits
  - to differentiate between myeloma (isotopic 'cold' areas frequently) and cystic secondaries (not frequently 'hot' centrally)

6. Bone density measurements

- with standard bone radiographs and densitometric scanning X-rays of progressive sclerosis of vertebrae **(74)**
- using a source of gamma rays which scan across a bone to give an absorption index of the density across the cortex and medulla
- computerised axial tomography (CAT scanning) used to measure the absolute amount of calcium per area of bone, **(75)** showing metastases

74 Progressive sclerosis of vertebrae

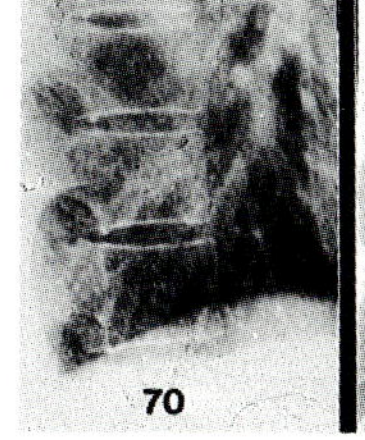

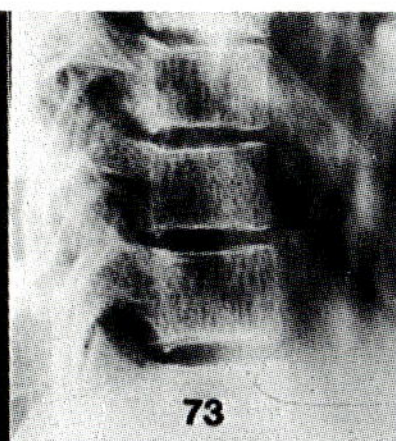

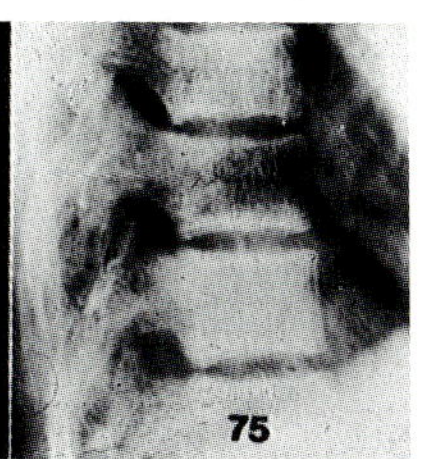

75 Metastases (CAT scan) – white masses in rami

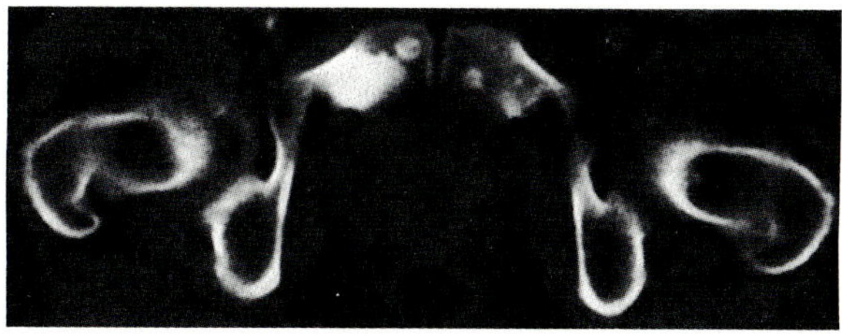

c. Investigation of the microscopic structure of bone

1. Normal bone

Bone consists of an organic matrix, osteoid, in which crystals of bone mineral hydroxyapatite are laid down (**76**). Osteoid is a protein and mucopolysaccharide ground substance containing collagen fibres. The hydroxyapatite crystals impart rigidity to bone and by ionic exchange through the cellular population maintain an equilibrium between the bone and blood content of calcium. The osteocyte and osteoblast are responsible for the simultaneous excretion of the protein matrix and the crystal nuclei which make up the two elements of bone (**77**). Usually calcification of the matrix shown as a calcification front keeps pace with the production of osteoid leaving a small rim of osteoid (**78** *fluorescent microscopy* × *200*). Up to the age of 60 years about 80 per cent of the bone osteoid surface is associated with a potential calcification front.

76 Calcification process

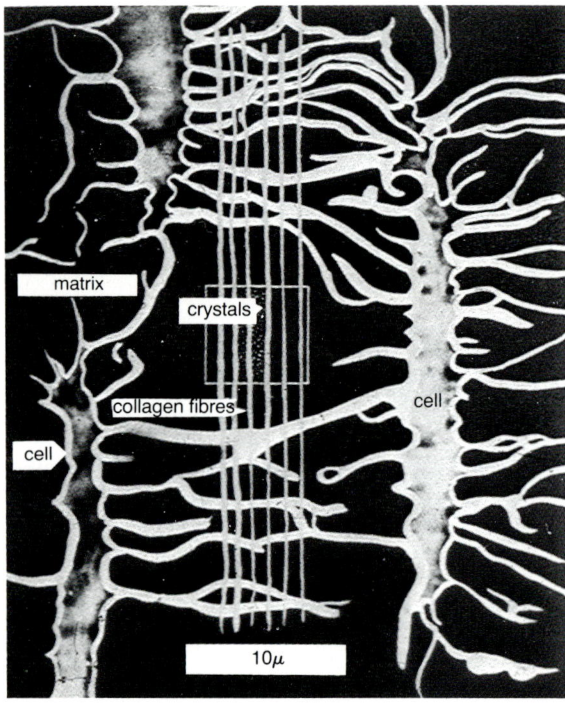

77 Cellular calcification mechanisms

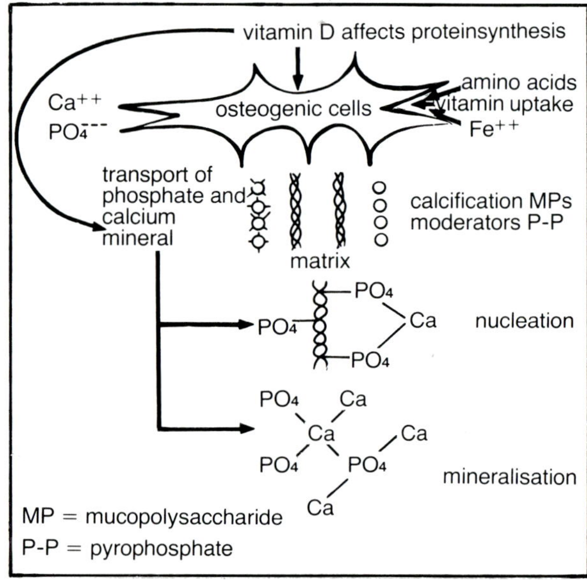

78 Rim of osteoid after tetracycline labelling

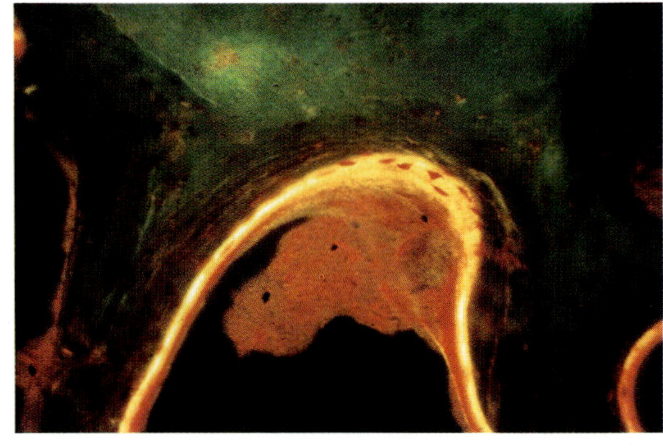

2. Quantitation of the metabolic status of bone

Iliac crest bone is commonly used in the diagnosis of bone disease. Quantitative measurement enables not only a diagnosis to be made but also an assessment of the severity of the disease and its eventual response to treatment. The biopsy is taken in a standard fashion (**79**) and preserved from deformation. The ideal site for biopsy is shown in **80**. A large trephine is used (**81**) so that a cylinder of bone is obtained which includes outer and inner tables of compact bone. Premedication and local anaesthesia are necessary, and the soft tissue and periosteum are cut and displaced before trephining.

The bone sample is fixed for 24 hours in 4 per cent formaldehyde which has been alkalised with sodium barbitone, or 70 per cent alcohol. Either two cores are taken or the cylinder of bone is carefully divided lengthways with a fine saw. The two parts are embedded separately for the preparation of mineralised and demineralised sections. Mineralised 6 μ sections are prepared from double resin embedded blocks (**82**).

79 Iliac crest biopsy

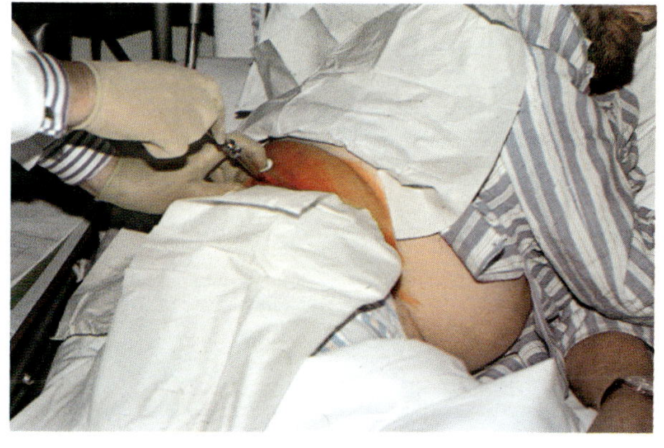

80 Site for transiliac biopsy

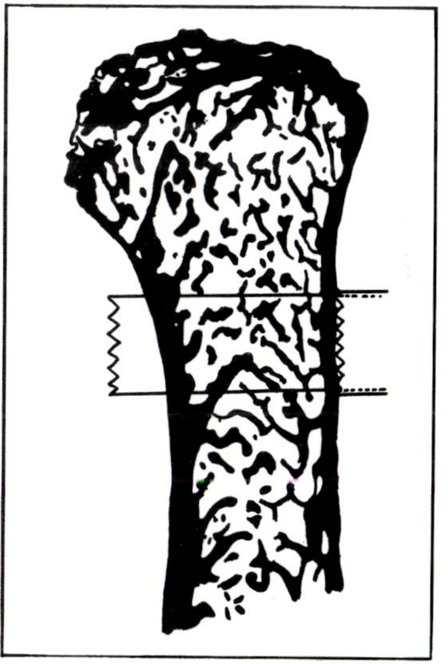

81 Bone trephine, 8 mm

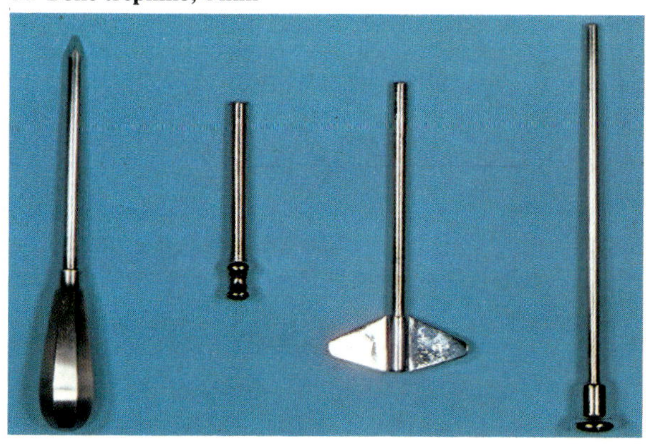

82 Resin embedded biopsy

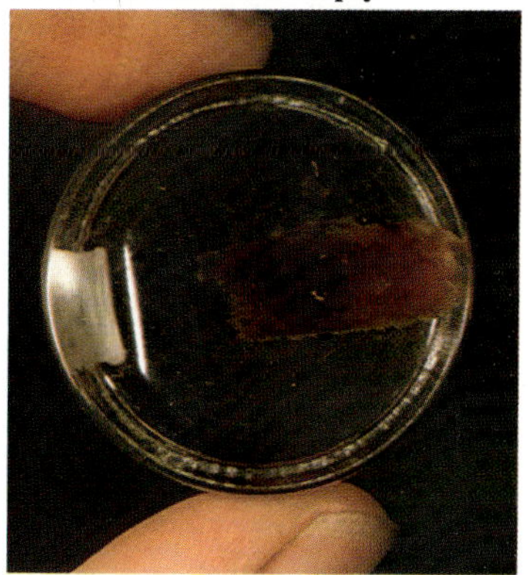

Bone sections are then processed in a variety of ways:

- demineralised sections are prepared to show the fine cellular structure and for an appreciation of the marrow (**83** *H&E* × *25*)
- mineralised sections
  - mineralised bone (black) and osteoid (brown) stained by von Kossa's method are shown in **84** (× *25*)
  - mineralised bone (blue) and osteoid (orange) stained by Goldner's method are shown in **85** (× *300*)
- scanning electron microscopy (SEM) to study the finer structure of bone surfaces, (**86** × *1800*)
- quantitative microradiology shows up the differing densities of recently mineralised bone (grey) and more densely mineralised bone (white), a 36 year old osteoporotic female (**87**)
- fluorescent microscopy of labelled bone. With prior labelling *in vivo* and less frequently *in vitro*, newly laid down bone will take up tetracycline and other pigments. This method is used to estimate the rate of apposition of new bone by measuring either the width of the label (**88** *fluorescent microscopy* × *450*) or more reliably the distance between serial labels

83 Cortical bone and marrow

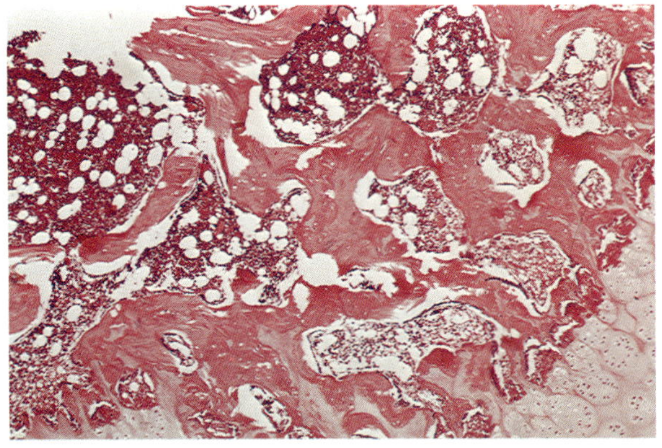

84 Osteomalacia – mineralised bone and osteoid

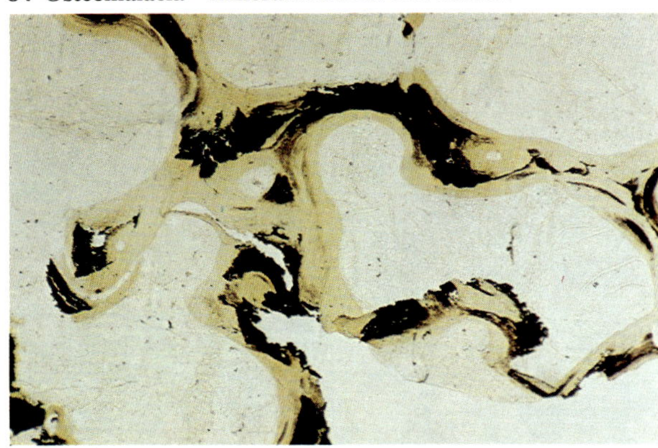

85 Mineralised bone and osteoid

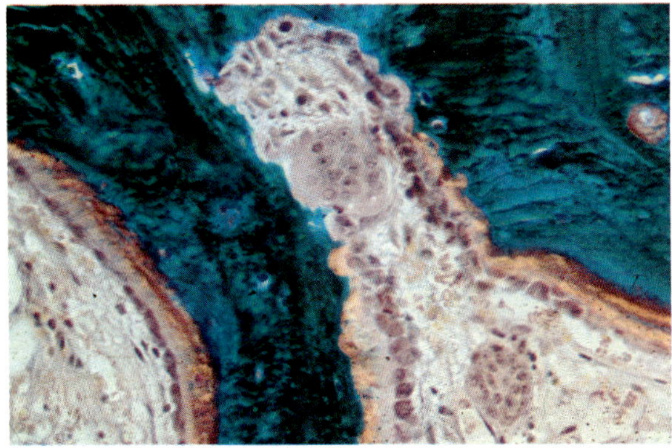

86 SEM of alveolar bone

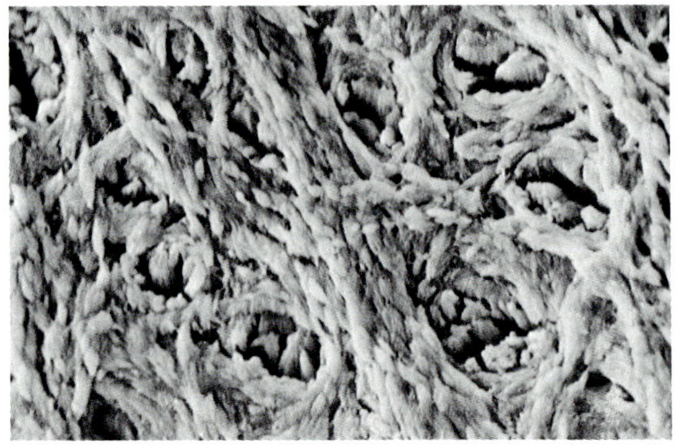

87 Microradiograph – osteoporotic bone

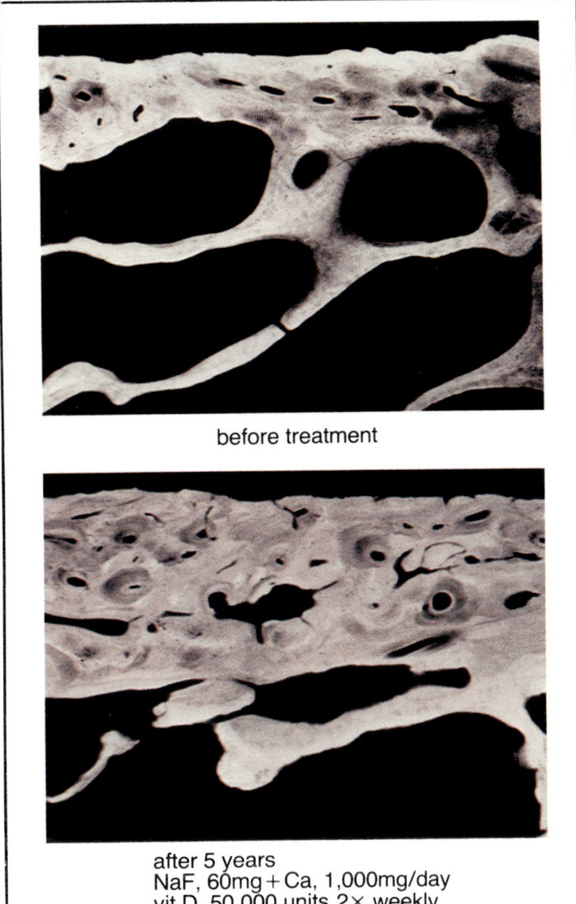

88 Tetracycline in newly formed bone

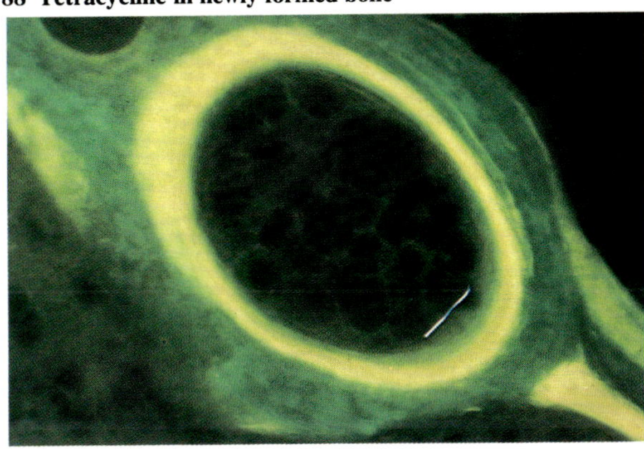

3. Quantitation using microscopy

Quantitative histology determines the amount of mineralised and non-mineralised bone in a given sample. A representative sample of cancellous bone is scanned either with a graticule (**89**), or by using an image intensifying system. The section is moved in stages under the graticule and the number of units on intersections of marrow, mineralised bone, osteoid etc is recorded. From this the ratio and percentage of each component can be calculated. This technique of point counting gives accurate results to within about 5 per cent.

89 Graticule on mineralised bone section

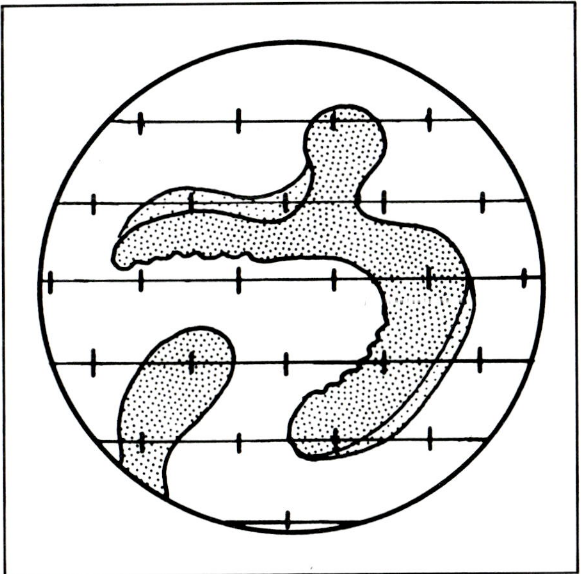

The total bone mass of the normal adult shows individual variation within a fairly constant range with a relationship to age (**90**). From adolescence to 50 years the mean is 22.79 per cent of the measured area. Over 50 years the mean falls to 15.5 per cent. Some of the lowest values, 5.5 per cent to 16.4 per cent (mean 8.9 per cent), are found in elderly women in the seventh to ninth decades (**91**).

In normal controls osteoid is patchily distributed over short lengths of trabeculae and accounts for only about 0.1 per cent of the areas measured.

Using these techniques a composite picture of normal and diseased bone can be built up. Bone is seen both as a skeletal structure undergoing constant renewal and as a metabolic store of ions such as calcium and phosphate which can be mobilised for healing fractures, foetal growth, lactation, muscle contraction and in times of mineral deprivation.

90 Bone density variations in males

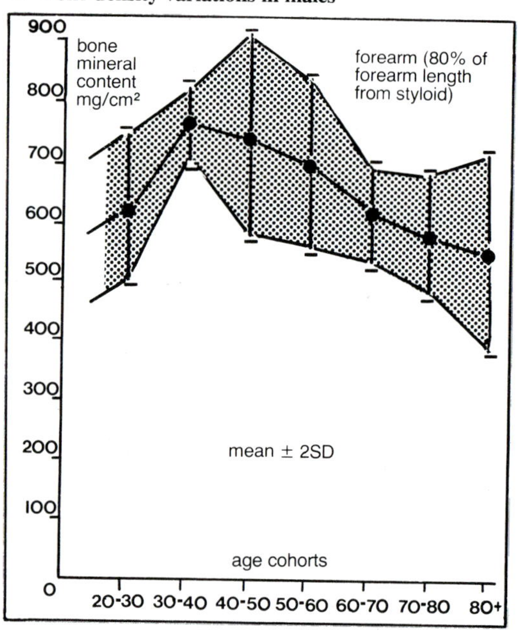

91 Bone density variations in females

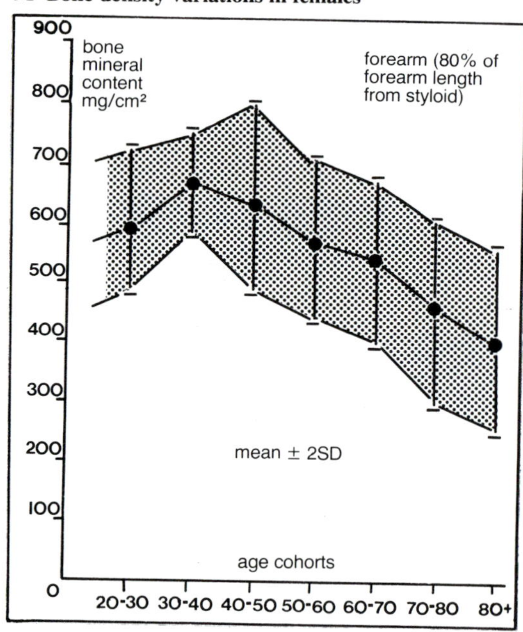

4. Cortical and cancellous bone

Cortical and cancellous bone is seen to consist of lamellae of bone when examined under polarised light (**92**). In the cortex the lamellae are arranged in concentric rings around a central canal containing blood vessels (**93**). Each unit in this branching structure is referred to as an osteon or haversian system (**94**). The spongy cancellous bone consists of trabeculae of parallel lamellae. The trabeculae are arranged to withstand stress, for example in the femoral neck (**95** and **96**).

Rapidly formed new bone in the foetus, at a fracture site or in Paget's disease is described as woven bone, a reference to the haphazard arrangement of the collagen fibres when viewed by polarised light (**97**). Woven bone eventually undergoes resorption and replacement by lamellar bone (**98**).

92 Bone lamellae under polarised light

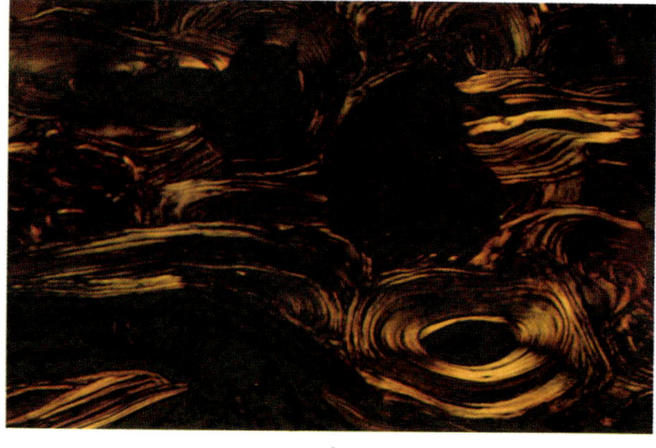

93 Central canal containing blood vessels

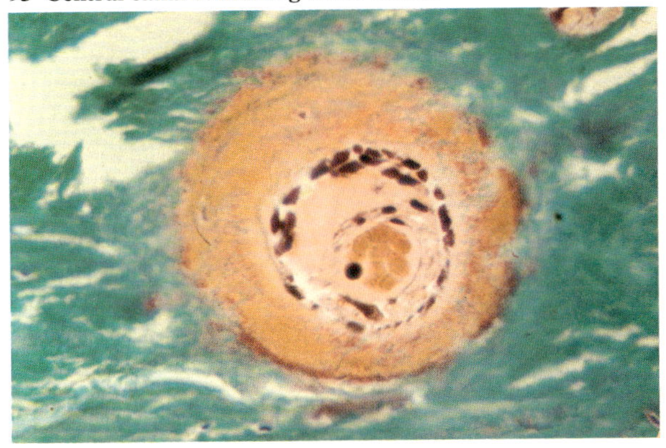

94 Haversian system

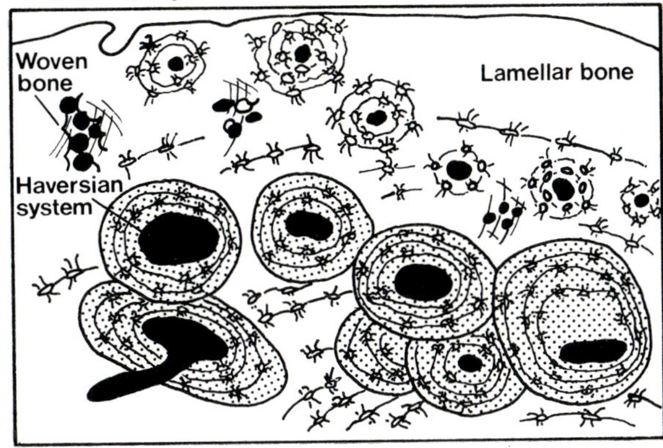

95 Fine structure of bone, trabeculae

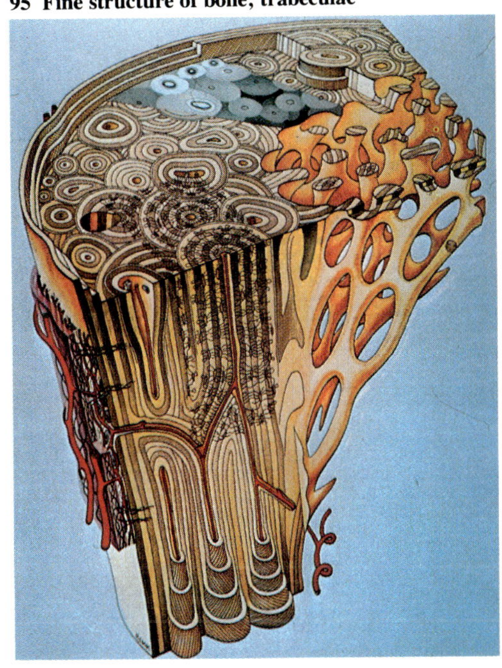

96 Mineral structure of bone, trabeculae

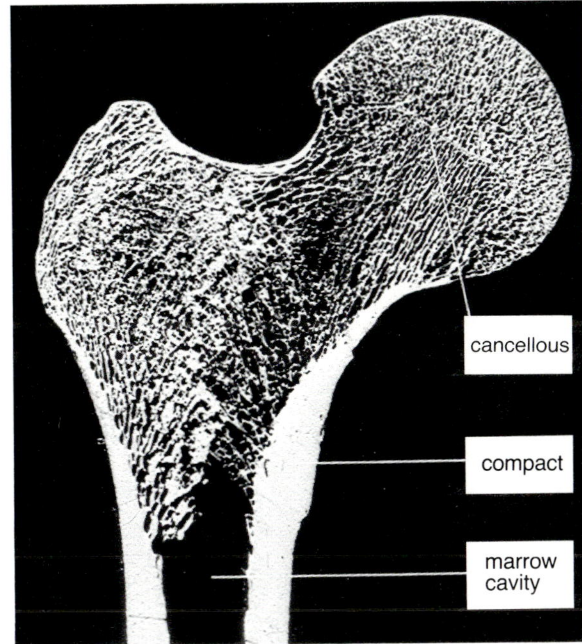

97 Woven bone

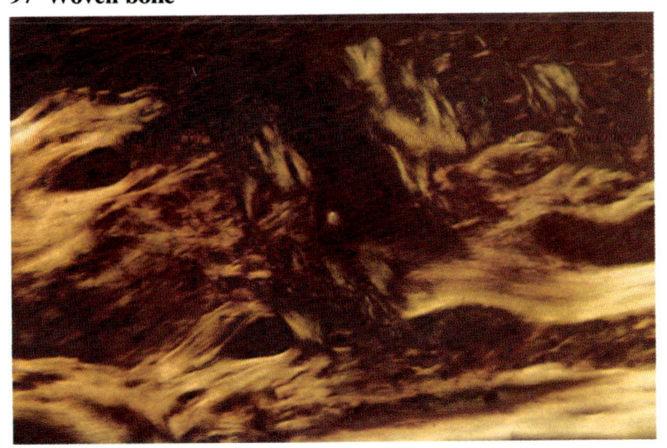

98 Lamellar bone

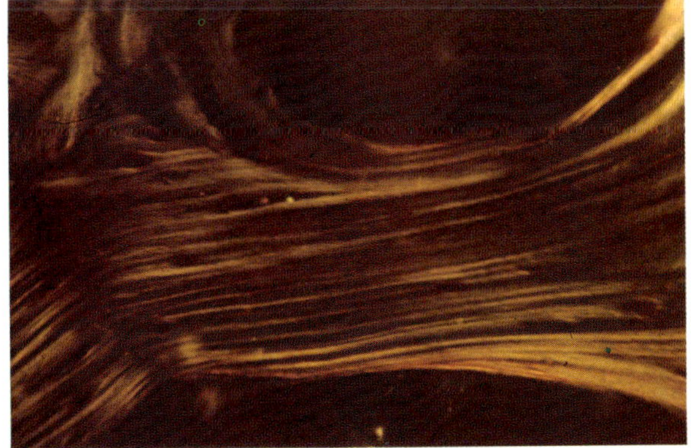

5. Bone formation

Long bones are formed by endochondral ossification. Cartilage consists of a gell of water and acid mucopolysaccharides, such as chondroitin sulphate, combined with non-fibrous proteins and fibrous proteins including collagens and elastin. The cartilage model grows by appositional growth exteriorly and by interstitial growth down the length of the shaft.

Ossification follows the differentiation of cells of the perichondrial membrane, a connective tissue sheath covering the bone, into osteoblasts. This occurs in mid-shaft and at both ends of the cartilage model. The epiphyseal plates remain cartilaginous until the bone is fully grown when the three areas unite and the plates ossify.

Flat bones such as the skull and sternum are first formed as connective tissue membranes. Mesenchymal cells forming the membrane are transformed into osteoblasts. These lay down osteoid which is then mineralised.

6. Bone cells

The principal bone cells are the osteocytes, osteoblasts (of varying maturity I–IV) and osteoclasts (**99**).

Osteoblasts rich in alkaline phosphatase form osteoid, the organic matrix of bone seen as a thin rim lining trabecular bone (**100** *Goldner's stain × 65*). They are readily identified by their single nucleus and close apposition to a trabecular surface (**101** *H&E × 250*). When active and closely applied to a growing seam of osteoid, osteoblasts are plump cells with basophilic cytoplasm.

99 Bone cells involved in ossification

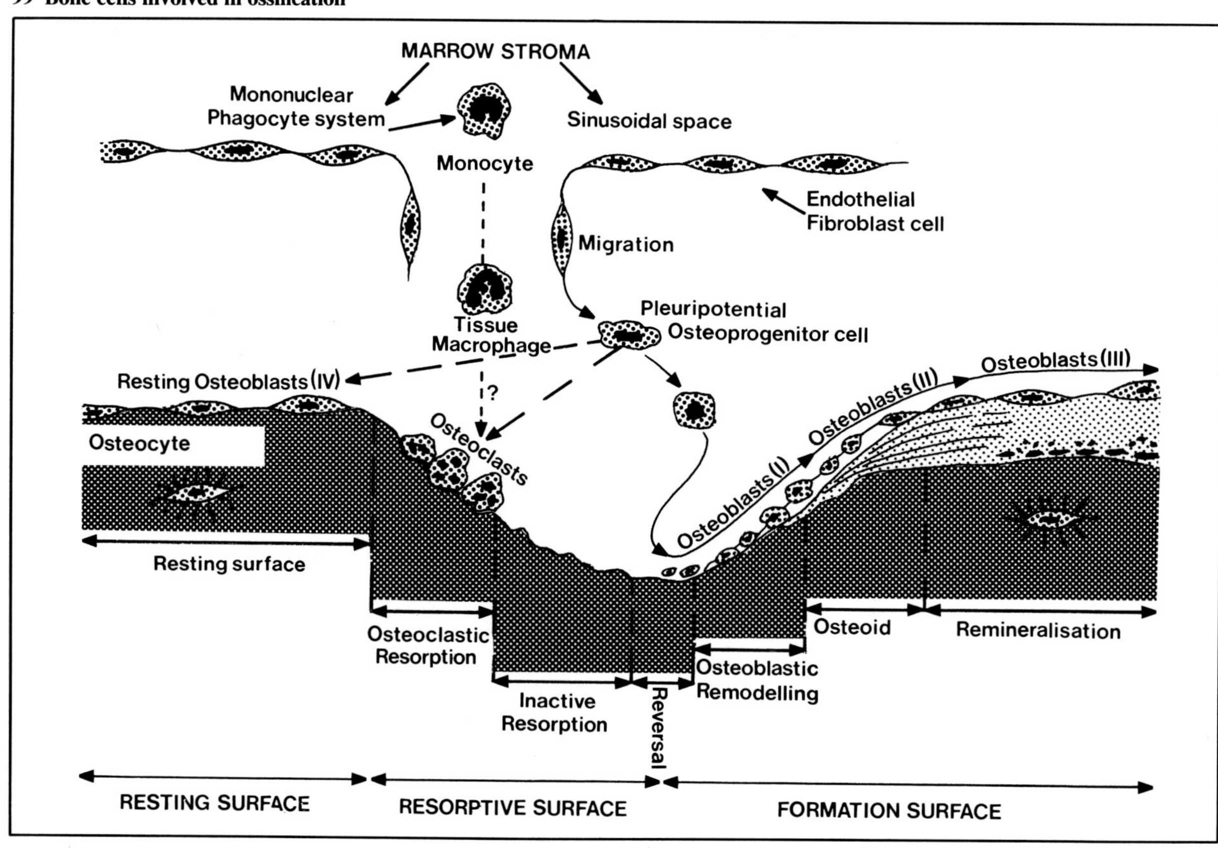

100 Osteoid seam covering trabeculum

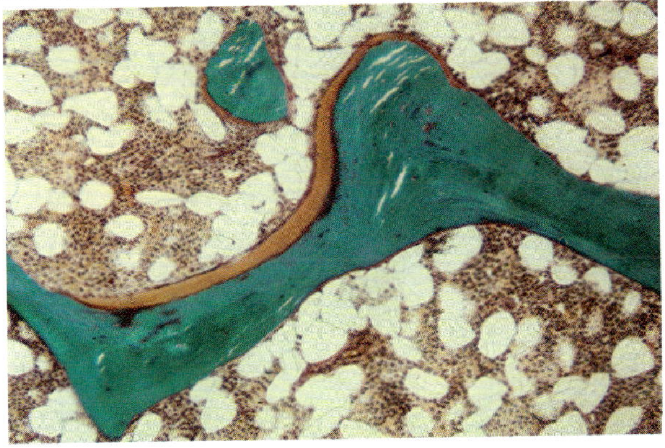

101 Plump active osteoblasts lining bone surface

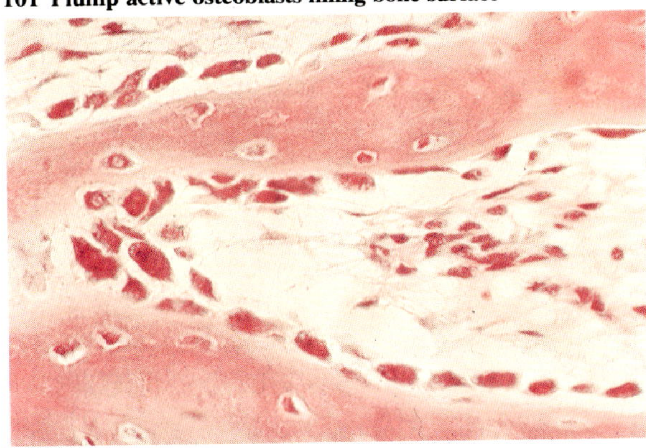

The resting osteoblast forming no osteoid is a slender cell applied to an almost invisible rim of osteoid on the surface of trabecular bone (**102** *H&E × 450*). Thus a complete sheath of cells separates the bone surface anatomically and metabolically from the rest of the body.

When an osteoblast becomes entrapped in the bone it is known as an osteocyte (**103** *basic fuchsin × 300*), its long spidery projections reaching into the bony lamellae. These cytoplasmic processes pass through canaliculi to form a syncytial network (**104** *basic fuchsin × 300*). Resorption of bone occurs around osteocytes, this process is termed osteocytic osteolysis in lumenae; the lumenae can then be remineralised, new matrix having been laid down in the middle of a trabeculum (**105** *H&E × 400*).

102 Slender resting osteoblasts lining bone surface

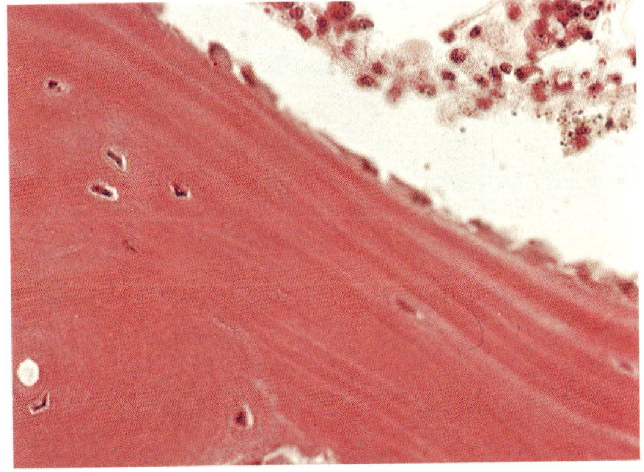

103 Osteocytes

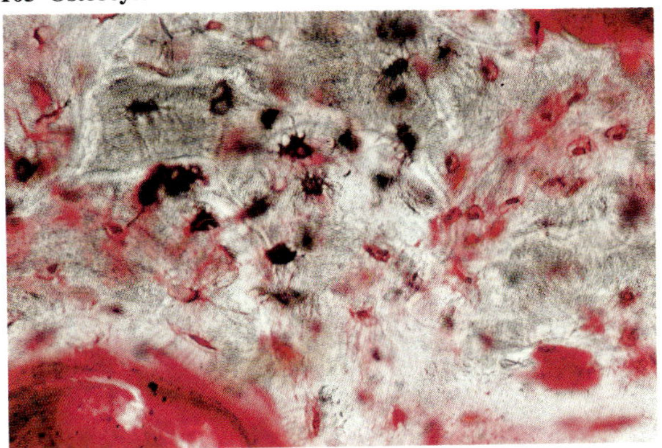

104 Syncytial network of osteocytes

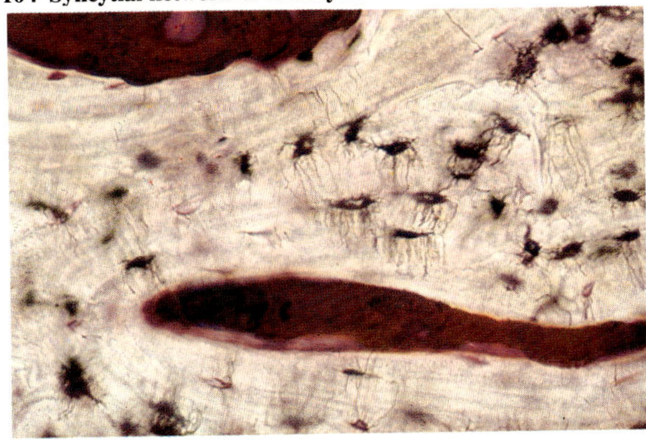

105 Osteocytic osteolysis

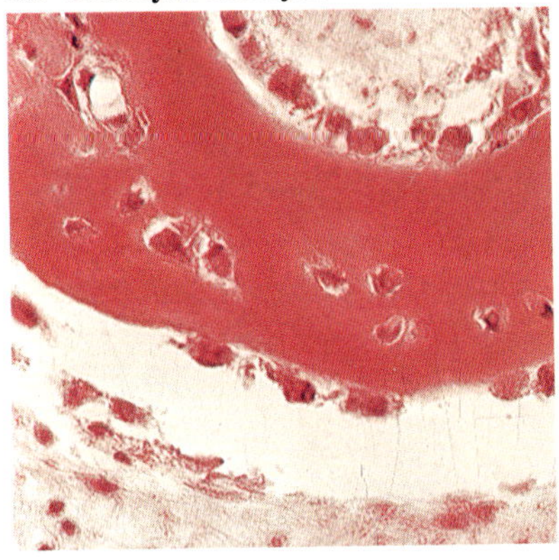

Osteoclasts are multinucleated giant cells which remove bone mineral and its matrix from the bone surface where they may be present in small clusters or singly. On the surface of bone undergoing resorption they are seen in small pits (Howship's lacunae) which they have eroded (**106** *H&E × 250*).

Osteoblasts and osteoclasts are usually found in close proximity (**107** *Goldner's stain × 200*). The mechanism of resorption may be particularly evident appearing as 'snail tracks' on scanning electron microscopy (**108**).

106 Howship's lacunae

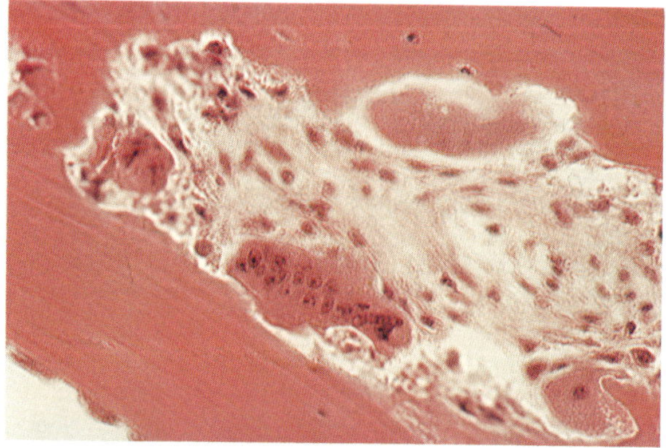

107 Osteoblasts and osteoclasts

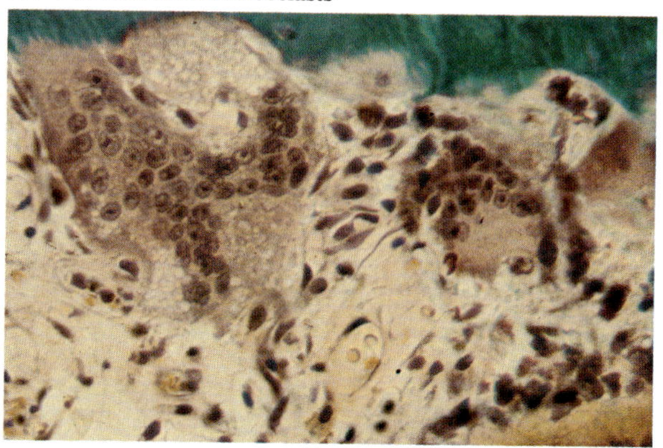

108 Osteoclastic tracks on bone surface

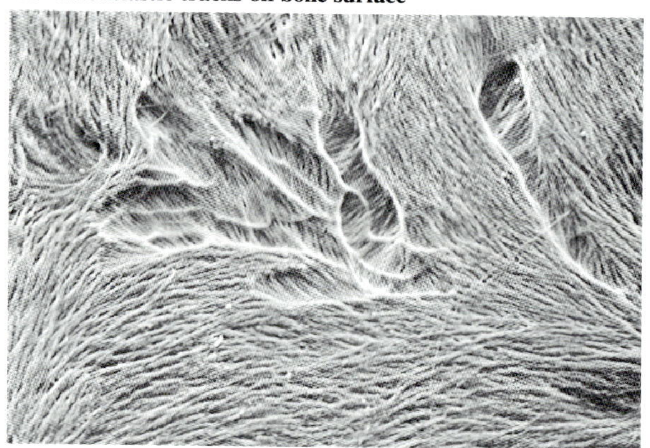

3. Metabolic and endocrine bone disease

Metabolic bone disease is largely a consequence of an upset in bone remodelling activity and/or mineralisation occurring at the periosteal, endosteal, haversian and trabecular surfaces.

Each centre of remodelling activity, of which there are millions, is derived from a collection of mesenchymal cells. These cells give rise to large multinucleated osteoclasts which resorb bone, and to osteoblasts which lay down osteoid (the organic bone matrix) and initiate mineralisation. Some osteoblasts persist as osteocytes and the remainder die. The sequence of events is invariable with resorption preceding new bone formation (**99**).

Mineralisation of seams of osteoid, laid down at bone surfaces by osteoblasts, involves the deposition of calcium and phosphate as hydroxyapatite crystals, measuring 30×2 nm, at so-called nucleation sites. These are situated at regular intervals along the collagen fibrils of the osteoid. The earliest deposition of calcium phosphate crystals can be detected as a fine nucleation front seen as a faint blue-brown line when stained by toluidine blue.

The five most important metabolic bone diseases are:

a. Rickets, clinical features shown in **109**
b. Osteomalacia, clinical features shown in **109**

Rickets and its adult equivalent osteomalacia have a variety of causes behind the common finding, at the cellular level, of a failure of mineralisation. Dietary vitamin D lack and poor solar irradiation, with failure of the synthesis of skin cholecalciferol, are the commonest causes. Failure of intestinal absorption, pancreatic and liver disease are often compounded with calcium and magnesium deficiencies. Phosphate or bicarbonate loss from the kidney or failure of the kidney to elaborate vitamin D are the mechanisms behind most renal rickets and osteomalacia. Other causes include anticonvulsant drugs and excessive use of diphosphanates or aluminium hydroxide.

109 Rickets and osteomalacia – clinical features

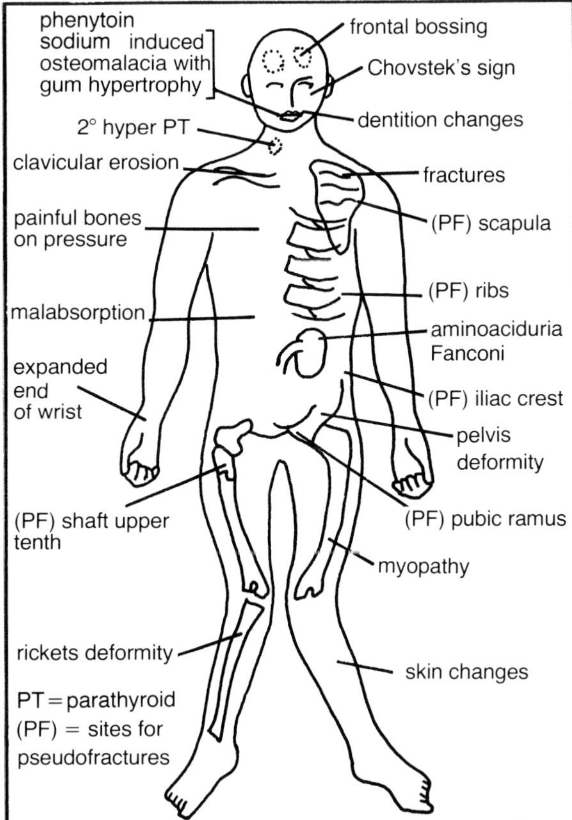

c. Osteoporosis, clinical features shown in **110**
d. Paget's disease of bone, clinical features shown in **111**
e. With the introduction of haemodialysis in the treatment of chronic renal failure, renal osteodystrophy has become increasingly important. It has features of osteomalacia, hyperparathyroidism, osteoporosis and osteosclerosis

110 Osteoporosis – clinical features

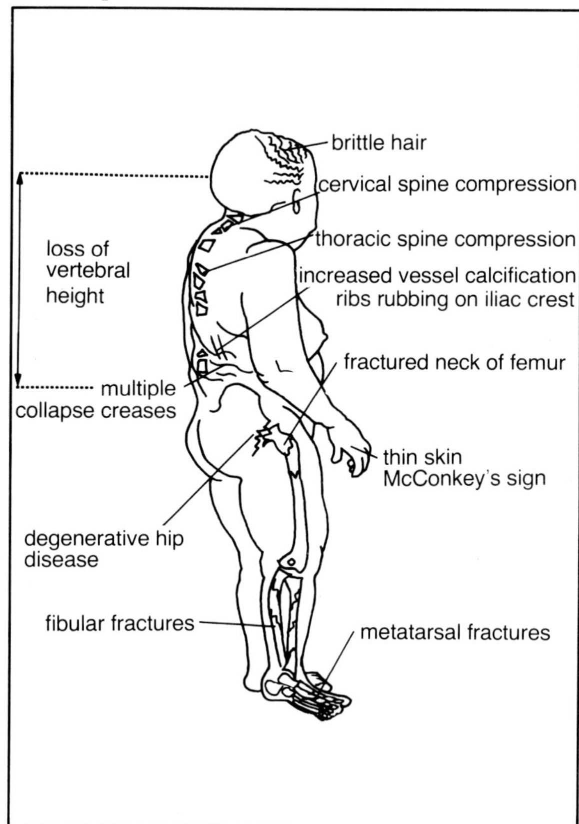

111 Paget's disease of bone – clinical features

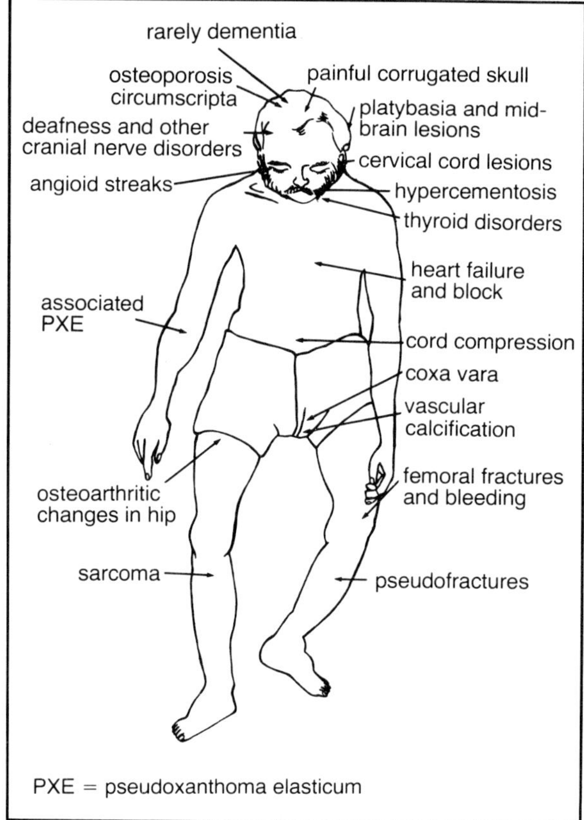

a. Rickets

Rickets is a metabolic disorder of childhood in which osteoid, the organic matrix of bone, fails to mineralise due to interference with calcification mechanisms (see **77**). The soft bones are prone to deformities.

Rickets is usually detected between the ages of 6 months and 2 years and in temperate climates is most common in dark skinned children. Weight bearing bones in the arms and legs show lateral and forward bowing (**112**). Generalised hypotonia linked with myopathy and lax ligaments is usual, resulting in a floppy baby.

The characteristic microscopic feature is an excess of osteoid present throughout the skeleton so that trabeculae of cancellous bone may consist of little more than osteoid (**113** *mineralised section, Goldner's stain × 150*). The osteoid is stained orange, the scanty mineralised bone blue.

Failure of mineralisation of the epiphyseal cartilages causes them to become thickened and irregular. The term 'rachitic rosary' is used to describe the enlargement of the costo-chondral junction.

The increased width in the rather disorganised epiphyseal plate is shown in **114** (*demineralised section, H&E × 150*).

In addition to deformities, the radiological appearances include widening and cupping (champagne glass appearance) of the distal ends of the long bones (**115**), increased space between diaphysis and epiphysis and poor mineralisation of the bones. Deformity and bowing of the ends of long bones (**116**) are further radiological features.

Bossing of the frontal and parietal bones is common. Wide sutures suggest a 'hot cross bun'. The anterior fontanelle may not close. The primary dentition may show enamel defects and caries and the permanent teeth hypoplasia.

112 Rickets

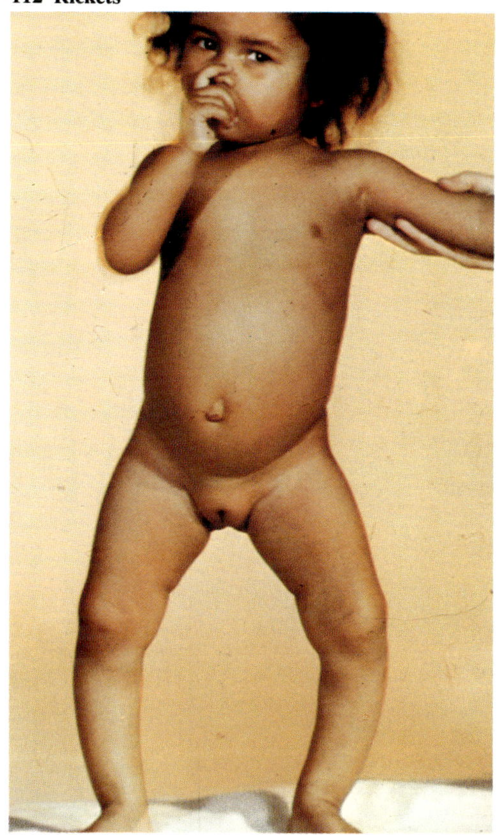

113 Rickets – excess of osteoid

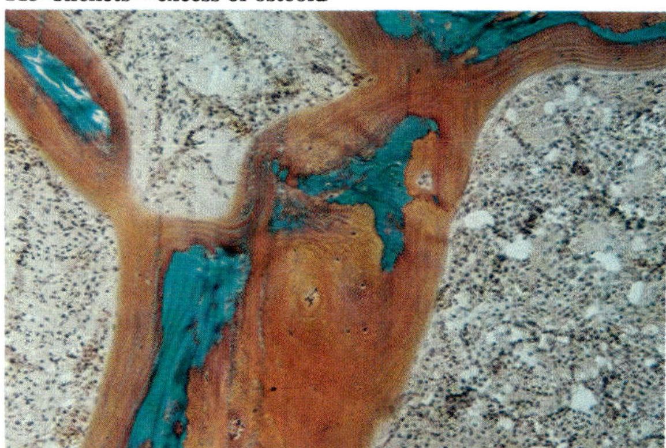

114 Rickets – disorganised epiphyseal plate

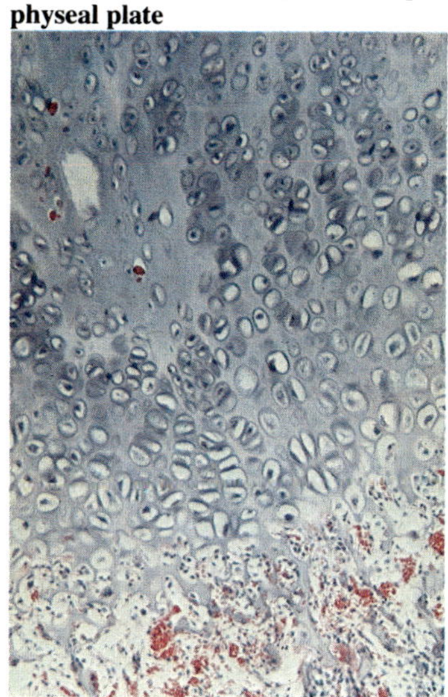

115 Rickets–champagne glass appearance

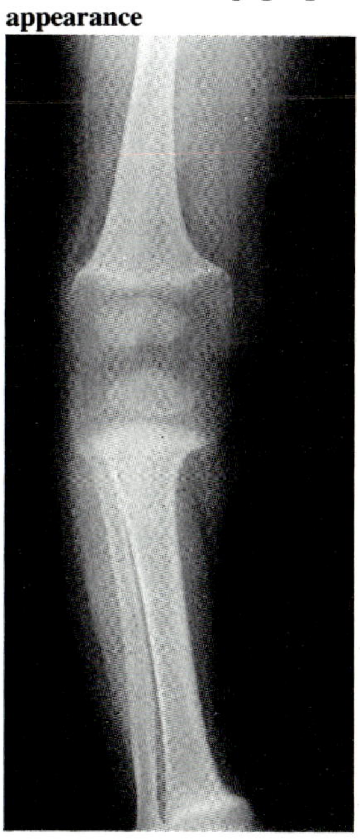

116 Severe rickets – bowing of long bones

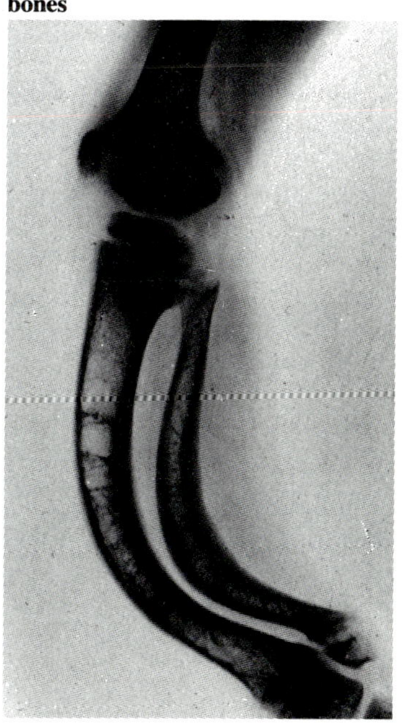

b. Osteomalacia

Osteomalacia is the adult counterpart of rickets and is characterised by failure of mineralisation and an excess of osteoid due to interference with calcification mechanisms (see **77**). The osteoid is increased at the expense of mineralised bone (**117**, **118**).

The diagnosis is established by bone biopsy and the examination of a mineralised section ground and stained by von Kossa's method which stains the mineral black/brown and leaves the osteoid unstained (**119** × *200*). Alternatively Goldner's method may be used which stains the mineralised bone blue and the osteoid orange (**120** × *360*). Both methods show a large excess of osteoid covering the trabeculae. Note the 6 lamellae in the top left hand corner of **120**. In normal bone the range is 0–3. They show up well with tetracycline staining (**121** *fluorescent light* × *200*).

A severe case of osteomalacia in a Pakistani female (**122** *Goldner's stain* × *150*), wife of the patient whose biopsy is shown in **120**. Their child had rickets. The mineralised section shows only a small quantity of mineralised bone which is stained blue.

The salient symptoms are bone pain and tenderness, a consequence of excessive deformation of the softened bones. The muscle weakness and characteristic gait frequently present could be due to depressed plasma calcium levels or vitamin D deficiency, both of which are related to contractability of muscle.

Radiographic features of osteomalacia include diminished bone density, loss of bone detail and the presence of Looser's zones which represent bands of unmineralised callus (osteoid), a result of small stress fractures and minor injuries. Arteriograms show Looser's zones in the upper shaft of the femur and in the pubic ramus occurring near vascular entry sites (**123** and **124**).

The classic severe case of osteomalacia with deformity of the skeleton seen as kyphosis, distortion of the ribs, bending of the pubic rami and fractures is uncommon (**125**). Fractures are slow to heal and remain painful for a long time because of deficient mineralisation.

117 Normal bone components

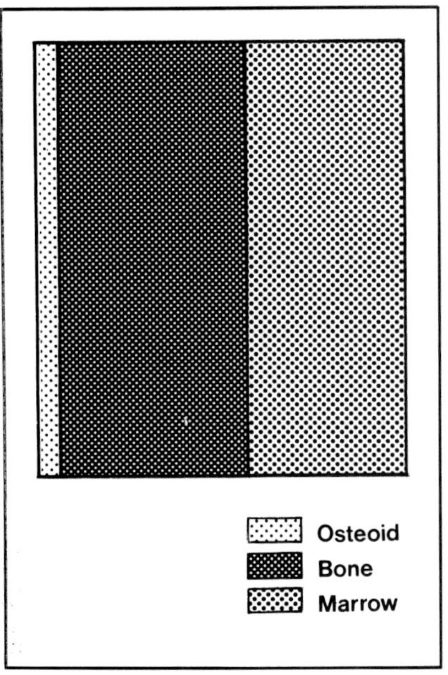

118 Osteomalacia – bone components

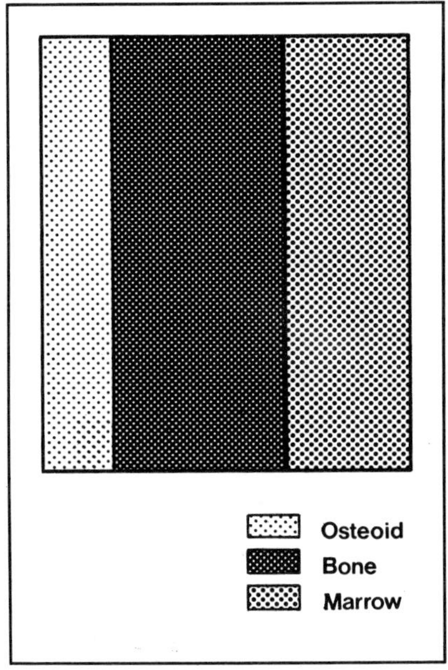

119 Osteomalacia – failure of mineralisation

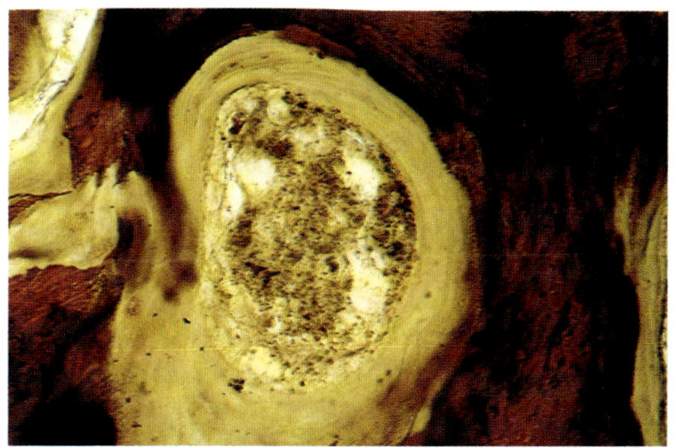

120 Osteomalacia – failure of mineralisation

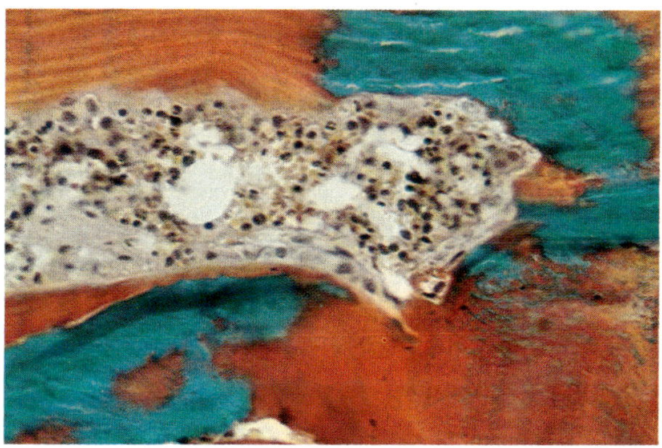

121 Osteomalacia – multiple lamellae

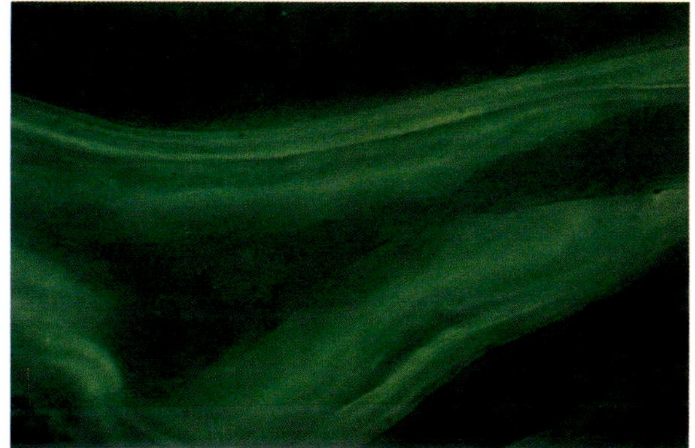

122 Nutritional osteomalacia

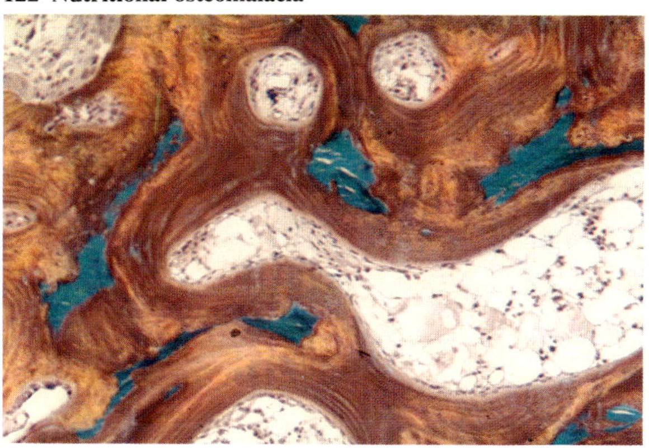

123 Osteomalacia – Looser's zones

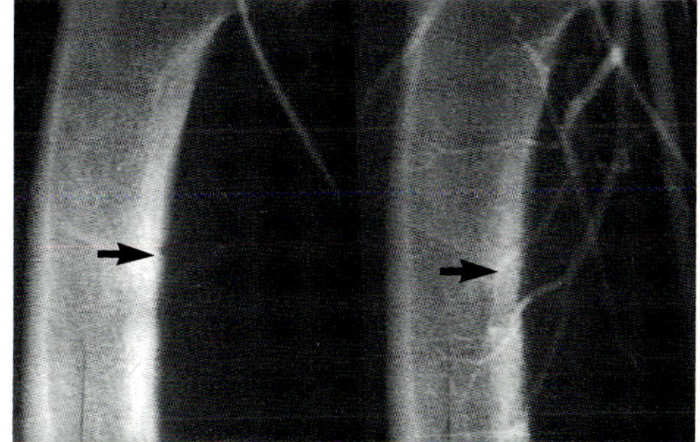

124 Osteomalacia – Looser's zones

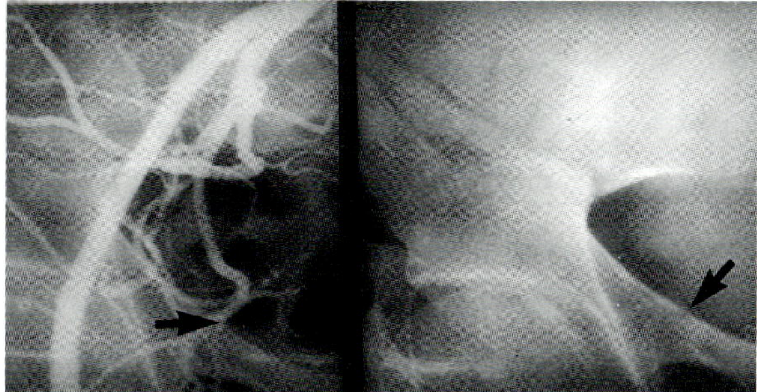

125 Severe osteomalacia

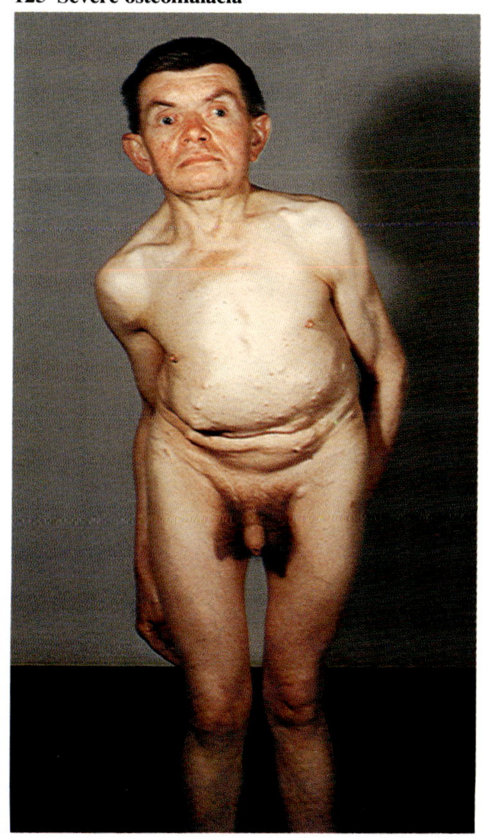

c. Osteoporosis

Osteoporosis is a decrease in bone mass resulting in thin fragile bones (**126**, compare with **117**).

In the head of the femur much of the compact bone is transformed into cancellous bone, and the trabeculae of the cancellous bone are reduced in number and thickness (**127**).

Cancellous bone in osteoporosis (**128** *mineralised section, von Kossa's stain* × *30*). The bone is fully mineralised but reduced in amount.

Osteoporosis is the commonest cause of pathological fracture. A common fracture site is the neck of the femur (**129**), the following sequence occurs frequently: a fall, leading to fracture of neck of osteoporotic femur, leading to deep vein thrombosis, leading to fatal pulmonary embolism.

A radiograph of severe osteoporosis affecting the humerus shows a loss of cortical thickness and an opening up of the trabecular pattern (**130**).

Compression and collapse of the vertebrae in severe osteoporosis (**131**). Chronic backache, bouts of severe back pain, loss of height and kyphosis are common complaints among osteoporotic patients. Skin creases appear and the ribs may rub on the iliac crest (**132**).

Osteoporosis and osteomalacia is a combination sometimes referred to as 'poromalacia' (**133**, compare with **117**, and **134** *von Kossa's stain* × *120*).

126 Osteoporosis – bone components

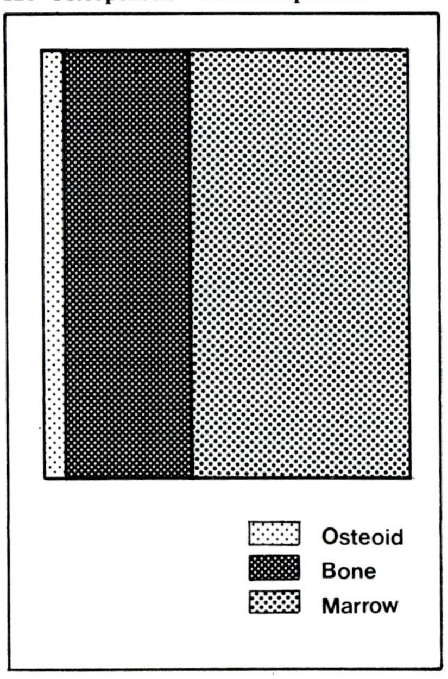

127 Osteoporosis – thin cortex and trabeculae

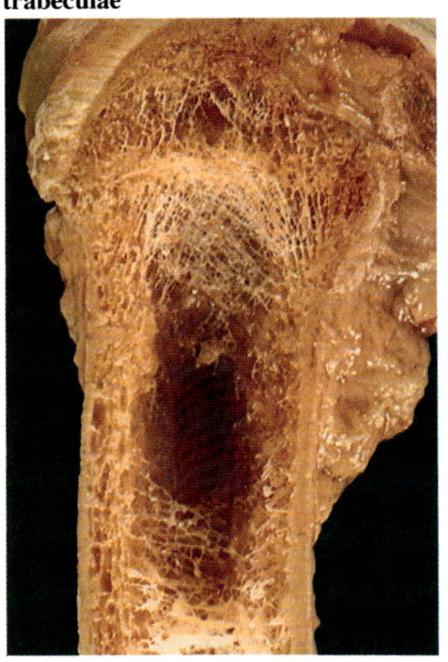

128 Osteoporosis – cancellous bone

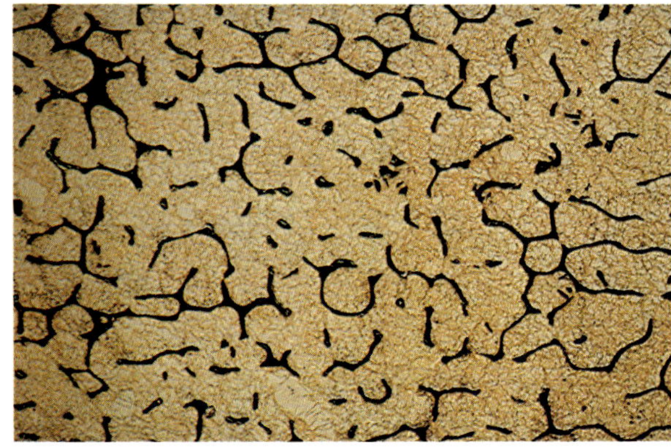

129 Osteoporosis – fractured femoral head

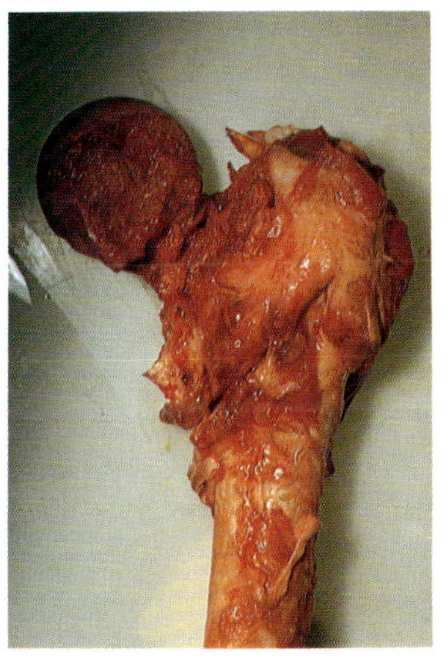

130 Osteoporosis in humerus

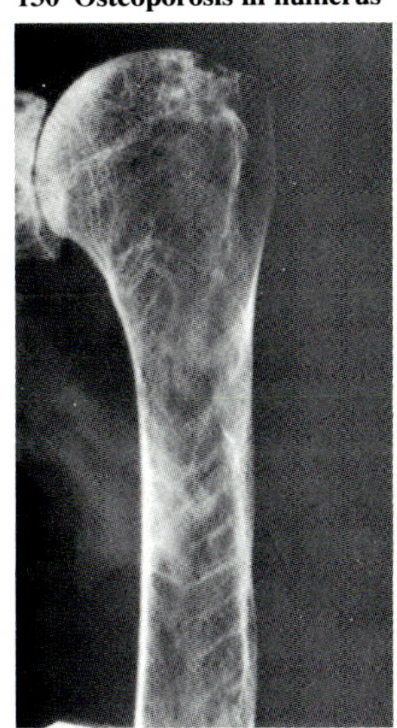

131 Osteoporosis – vertebral collapse

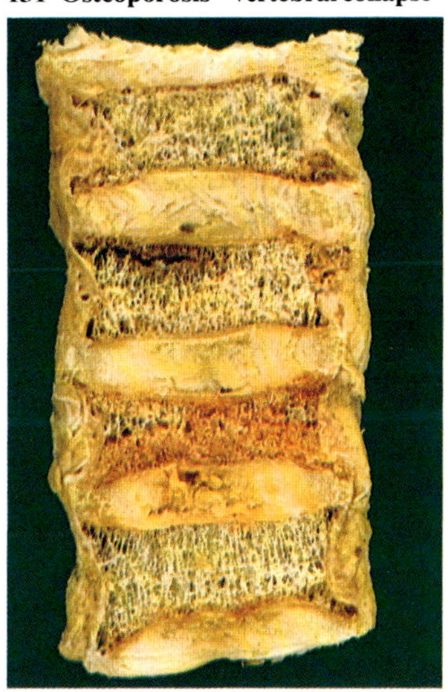

132 Osteoporosis

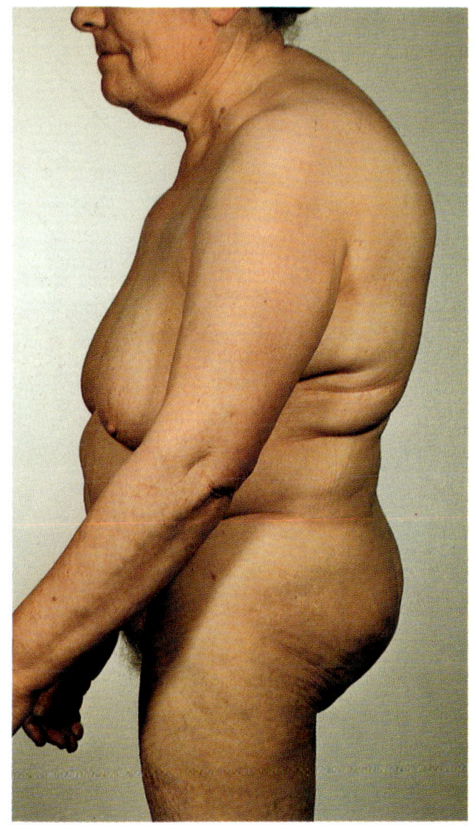

133 'Poromalacia' – bone components

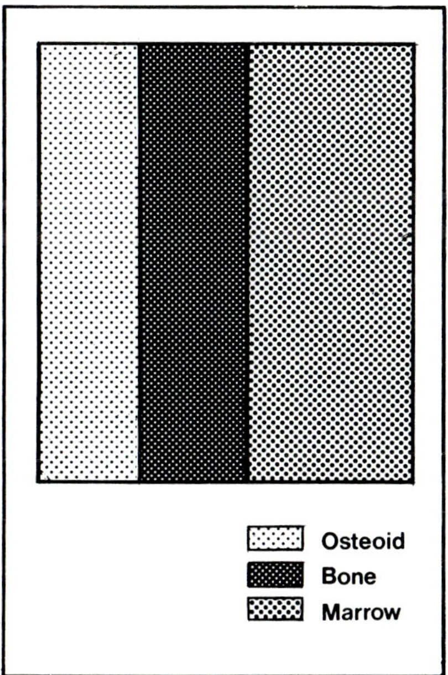

134 'Poromalacia' – trabeculae

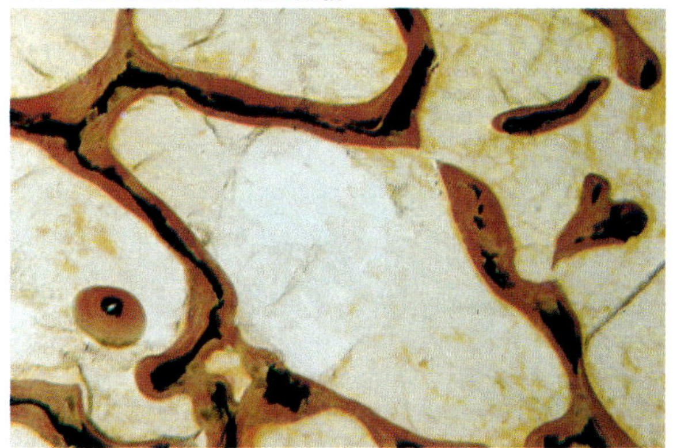

Osteoporosis is difficult to diagnose. The serum calcium, phosphate and alkaline phosphatase are usually normal. The pathological condition correlates well with radiology, particularly of the second metacarpal and the femoral head and neck region where grades of osteoporosis vary according to the visible trabecular pattern (**135**, numbers refer to the Singh index grading, and **136**). Iliac crest biopsy is the most valuable procedure and, if mineralised sections are prepared, will permit the diagnosis of co-existent osteomalacia.

Bone loss occurs in all women after the menopause but with great individual variation in rate. Mineralised sections of iliac crest bone from females aged 20 years (**137**) and 80 years (**138**) show the diminution of bone with ageing (*H&E × 150*).

135 Osteoporosis – sites of trabecular loss

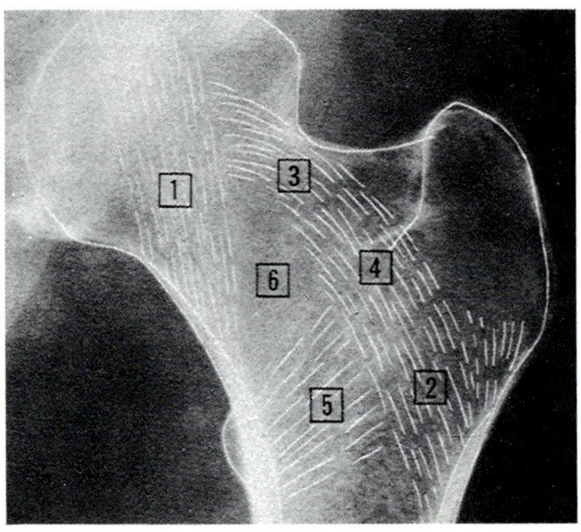

136 Osteoporosis – Singh index grading

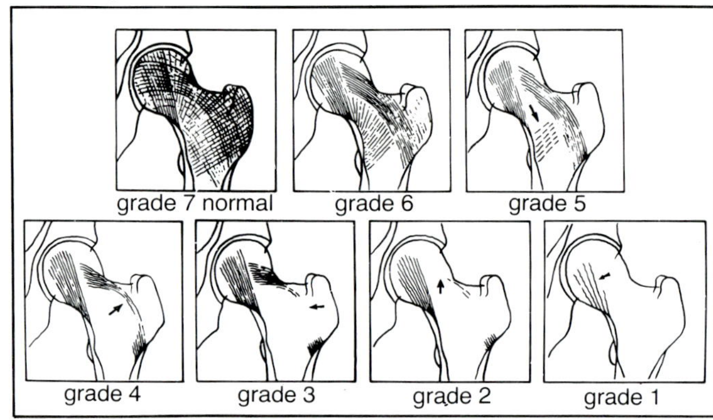

137 Normal bone trabeculae

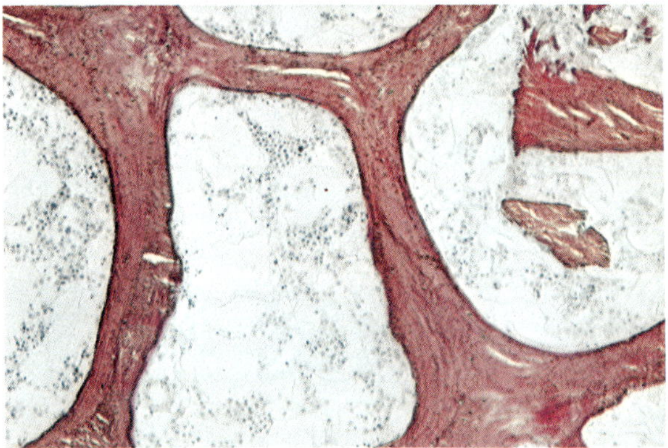

138 Thin bone trabeculae in osteoporosis

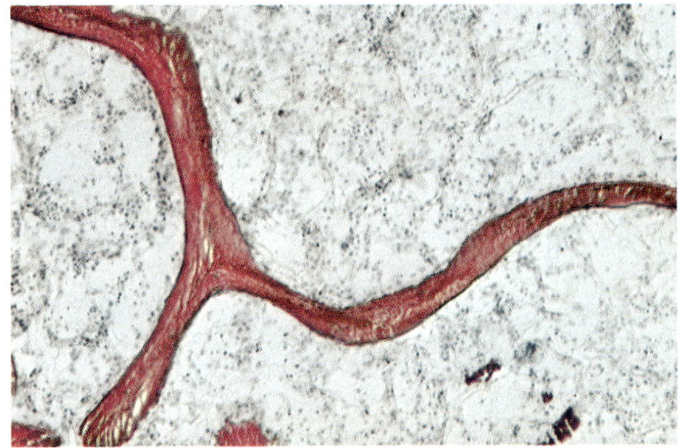

For practical purposes osteoporosis is classified according to its cause:

- senile or post-menopausal: most osteoporotic patients are post-menopausal women. Compare the vertebrae from females aged 20 years and 80 years (**139**)
- disuse osteoporosis: may be localised or generalised. Immobilisation of a limb will lead to localised osteoporosis (**140**). Prolonged bed rest, paralysis, physical inactivity and weightlessness of space flight can all lead to generalised osteoporosis
- Cushing's syndrome or prolonged corticosteroid therapy (**141**) both result in an increased urinary and faecal calcium excretion with a negative calcium balance resulting in osteoporosis. Note the pigmentation, truncal obesity and muscle wasting. Sections of the iliac crest show extreme porosity (**142** and **143** *demineralised sections H&E × 30*)

- changes in thyroid function have profound effects on the remodelling of bone: hyperthyroidism increases structural remodelling but with greater resorption than formation. The arm of a woman with thyrotoxicosis shows multiple fractures (**144**)
- sometimes the causation is multifactorial: for example a post-menopausal female may be immobilised by rheumatoid arthritis and treated with corticosteroids

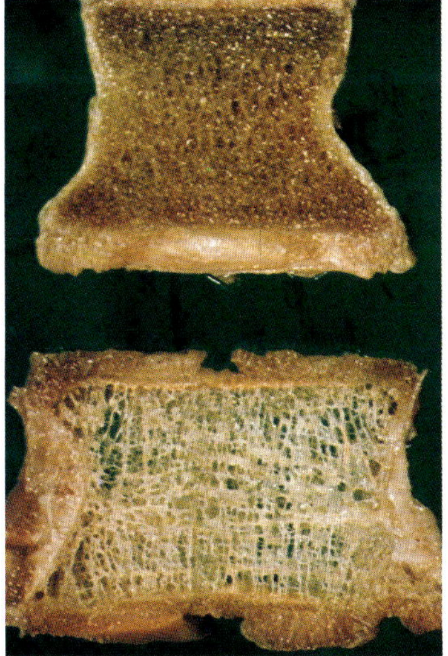

139 Senile osteoporosis

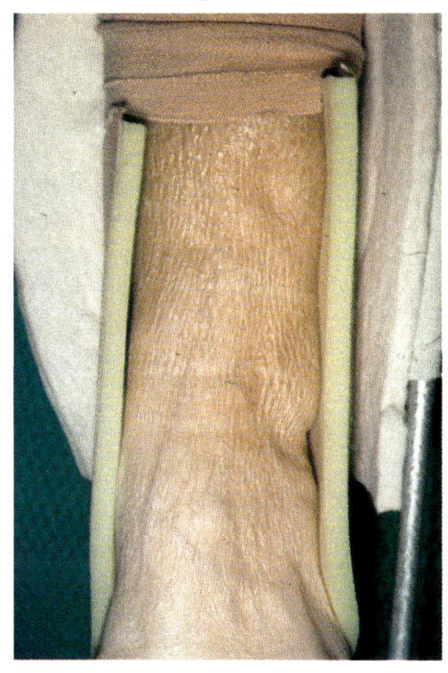

140 Disuse osteoporosis

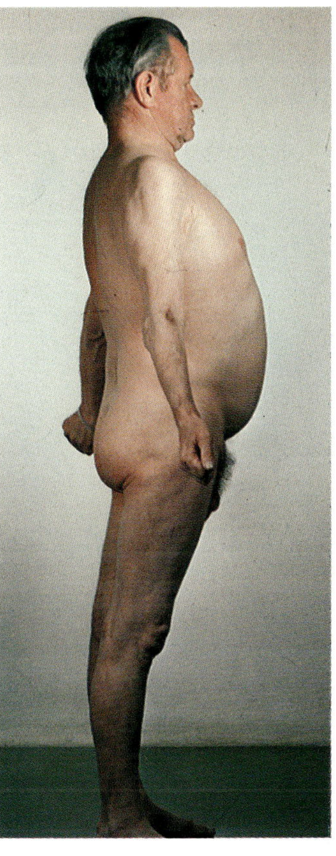

141 Steroid osteoporosis

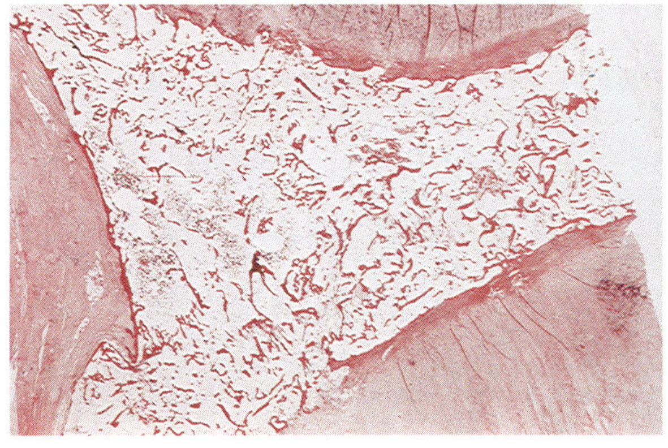

142 Cushing's disease/osteoporosis – whole section of iliac crest

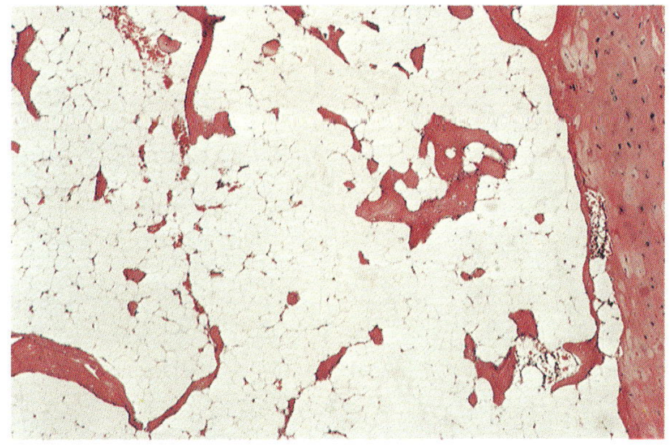

143 Cushing's syndrome – iliac crest biopsy

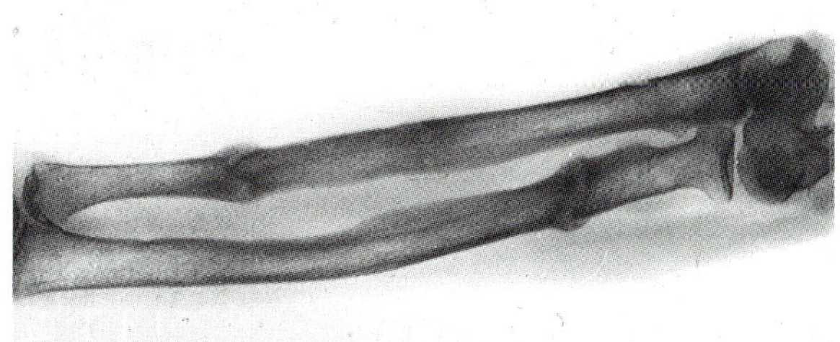

144 Osteoporosis in thyrotoxicosis

- transient osteoporosis (juvenile osteoporosis) in childhood affects a small group of apparently healthy children who become acutely osteoporotic. Recovery is the rule. The cause is unknown. A 16 year old boy with multiple osteoporotic fractures of the spine (**145**) showing kyphosis and chest deformity
- pregnancy osteoporosis is rare
- in cirrhotic liver disease and severe protein calorie malnutrition osteoporosis is frequent. The tibia and fibula show thinning in cirrhosis (**146**)

145 Juvenile osteoporosis

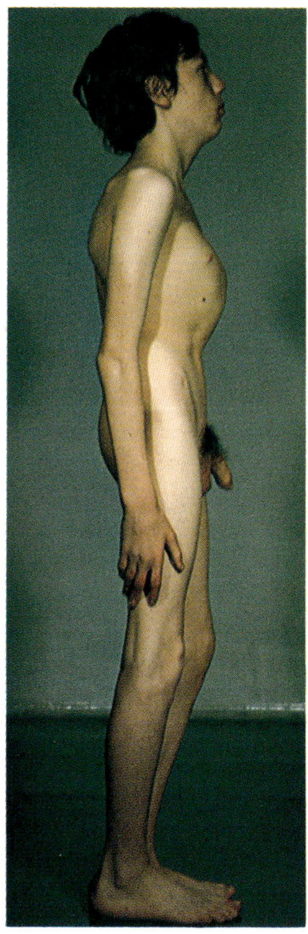

146 Osteoporosis in cirrhosis

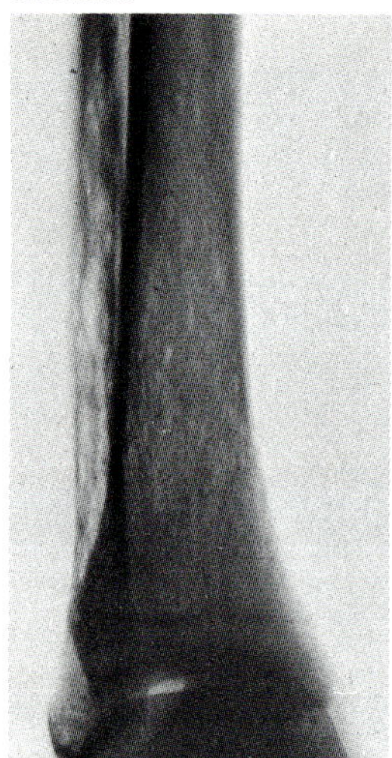

d. Paget's disease of bone

Paget's disease of bone originates from an upset in bone remodelling activity with irregular haphazard destruction of bone combined with excessive new bone formation. The cause is unknown but genetic inheritance and other connective tissue disorders are associated with the disease.

Sir James Paget's classic description of the advanced generalised bone disease that bears his name has never been bettered: 'It begins in middle age or later, is very slow in progress, may continue for many years without influence on the general health, and may give no other trouble than those which are due to the changes of shape, size, and direction of the diseased bones. Even when the skull is hugely thickened and all its bones exceedingly altered in structure, the mind remains unaffected. The disease affects most frequently the long bones of the lower extremities and the skull, and is usually symmetrical. The bones enlarge and soften, and those bearing weight yield and become unnaturally curved and misshapen.'

However, the name he suggested, osteitis deformans, is inappropriate because the condition is neither inflammatory, nor in its common monostotic form is it deforming.

The classic case of the rare severe generalised Paget's disease is that of a deaf old man with a bent back, bowed legs, curved tibia, a large skull and wobbling gait. The arms appear relatively long and the patient ape-like (**147** and **148**). Some patients with severe Paget's disease may have few complaints whereas others with a lesser degree of involvement suffer severe persistent pain.

147 Paget's disease affecting lower limbs

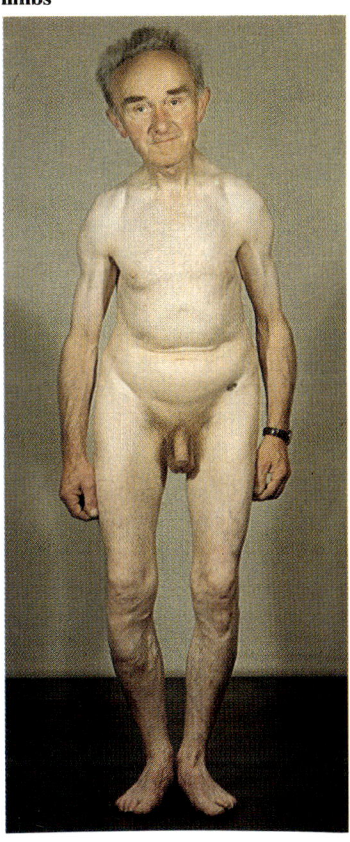

148 Paget's disease involving whole skeleton

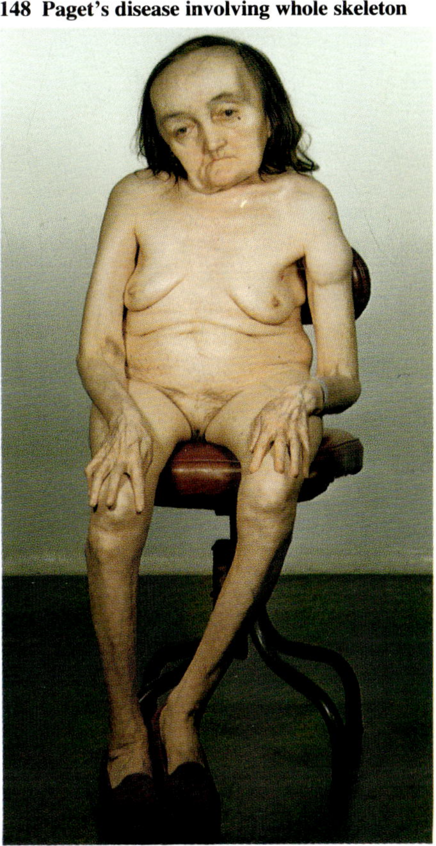

An isolated lesion affecting a single bone is not uncommon. Overall the disease is found in about 3 per cent of unselected hospital autopsies on individuals over 40 years of age. In this solitary lesion of the tibia the cortical and cancellous bone are thickened and there is a loss of demarcation between them (**149**). In long bones the process often starts at one end and advances along the shaft. Despite their solid appearance, the affected bones are poorly mineralised, translucent on X-ray (**150**) and readily deformed by weight bearing, showing microfractures (**151**).

149 Paget's disease – tibia

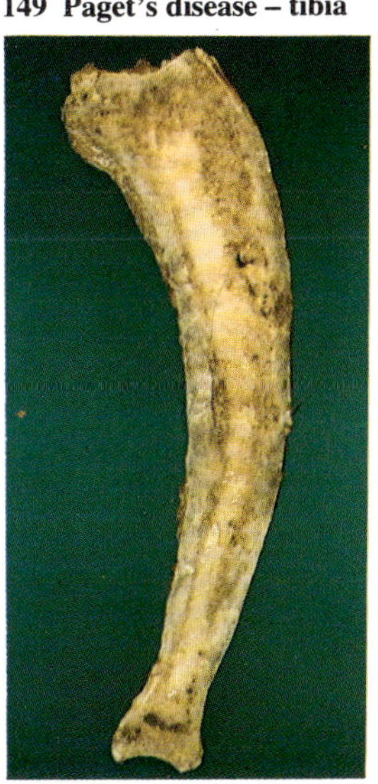

150 Paget's disease – tibial bowing

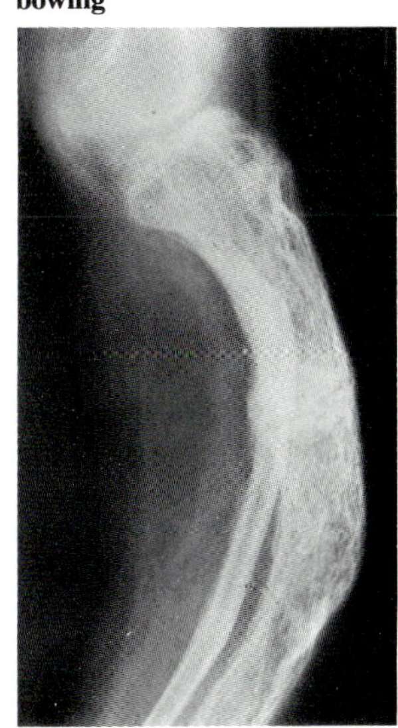

151 Paget's disease – microfractures

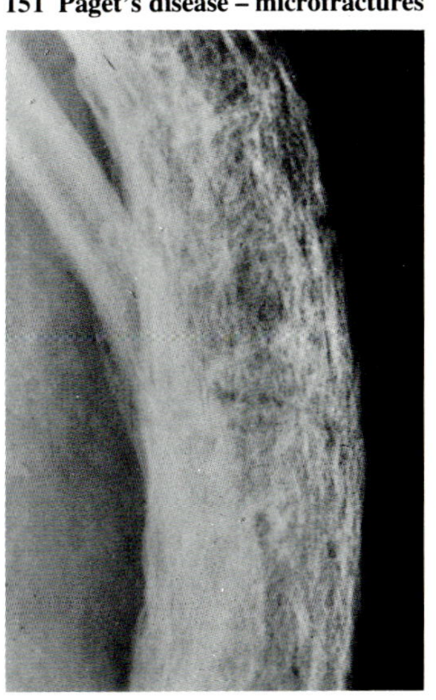

The initial bone lesion seen microscopically is osteoclastic resorption at the bone surfaces (**152** *mineralised section, Goldner's stain* × *200*). The pelvis, lumbar vertebrae, skull, femur and tibia are most frequently involved.

Osteoclastic resorption is followed by osteoblastic activity and the two processes are invariably seen together (**153** *mineralised section, Goldner's stain* × *350*). The large excess of osteoid results in soft, easily deformed bones. Pathological fractures are common. They may be incomplete (fissure fractures) or complete.

Random foci of newly formed bone are separated by 'cement lines' which indicate surfaces where bone resorption has been followed by deposition of new bone. They give a mosaic pattern, a characteristic diagnostic feature (**154** *demineralised section, H&E* × *150*). The marrow of the affected bone is replaced by cellular, extremely vascular, fibrous tissue. This increases blood flow through the bone so the affected part feels warm. Left ventricular hypertrophy and cardiac failure may result.

The randomly formed foci of new bone have a woven pattern when viewed by polarised light (as in foetal bone, fracture callus and renal osteodystrophy) (**155**).

152 Paget's disease – osteoclastic resorption

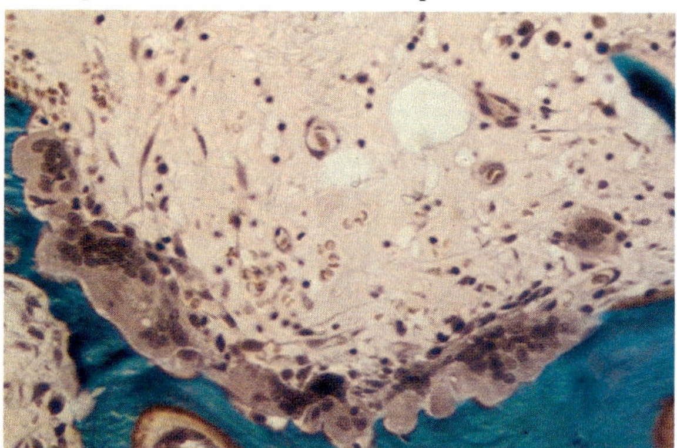

153 Paget's disease – osteoblastic activity

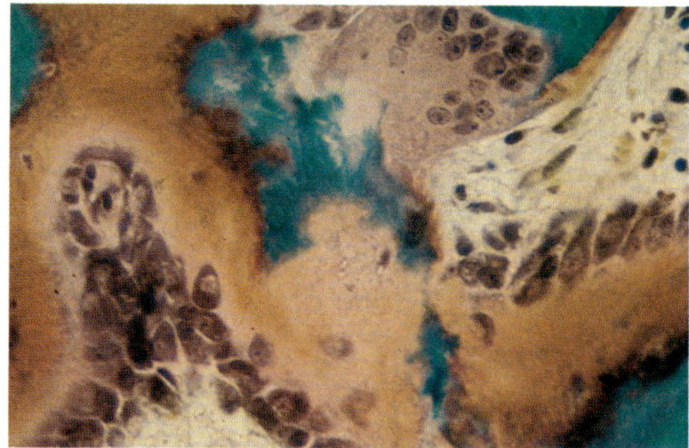

154 Paget's disease – mosaic cement lines

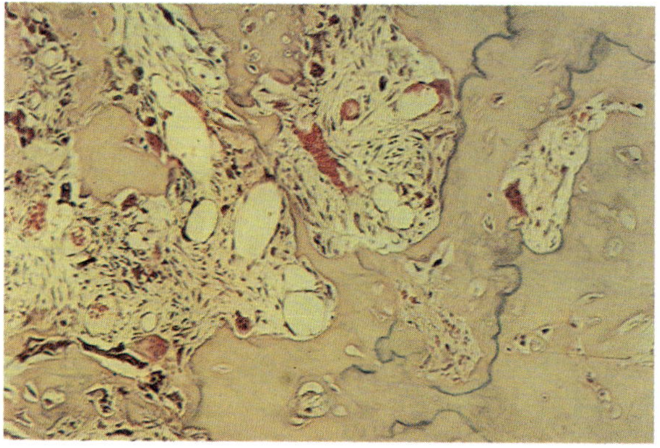

155 Paget's disease – woven bone pattern

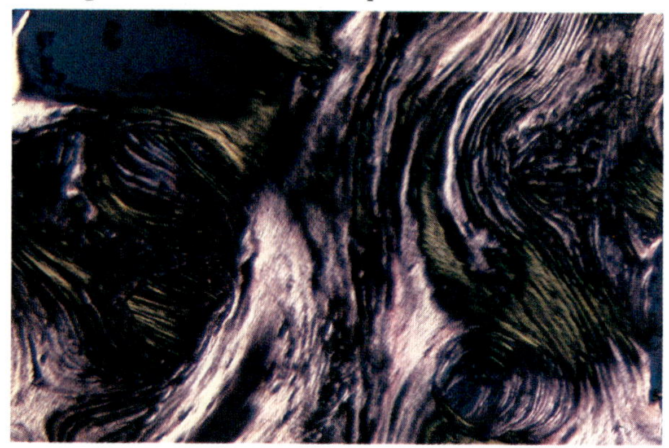

The skull when affected is grossly thickened and the sutures are obliterated (**156**). Occasionally at an early stage of the disease an area may be so rarefied as to suggest a bony defect (osteoporosis circumscripta **157**). Thickening of the skull may cause headache, deafness and loss of vision. Rarely, telescoping of the cervical vertebrae into the soft base of the skull (basilar invagination) causes cranial nerve lesions (see **159**).

156 Paget's disease – skull

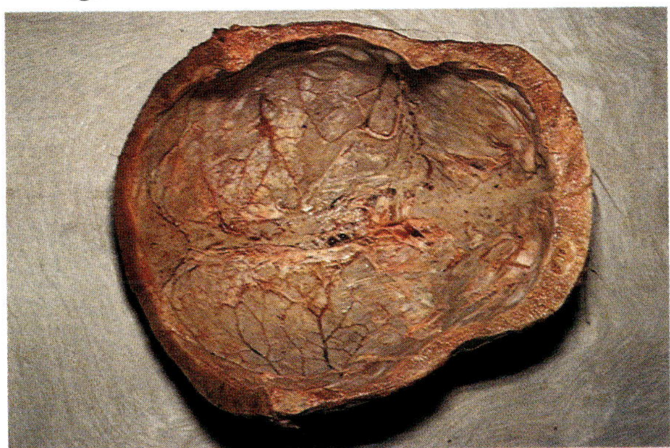

157 Osteoporosis circumscripta

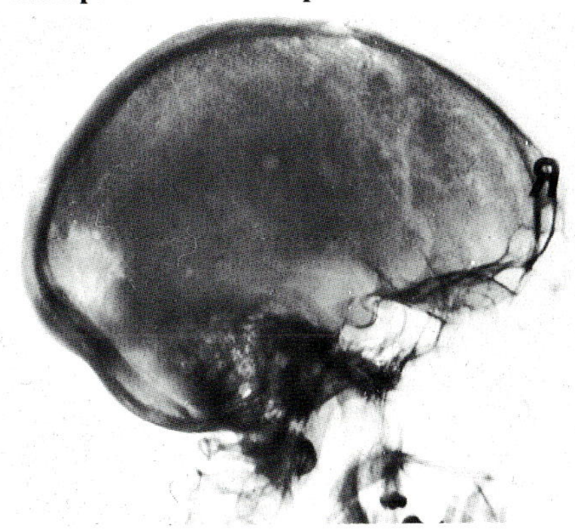

Many cases of Paget's disease are asymptomatic and the disease is often noted as an incidental radiographic finding. The characteristic features are:

- coarsening of the trabecular pattern shown in the femoral heads on radiograph (**158**)
- areas of apparent osteolysis, particularly in the skull (**159**)
- expansion of the bone in a concentric fashion, a 1000 year old skeleton found in Yorkshire (**160**)

158 Paget's disease – femoral head

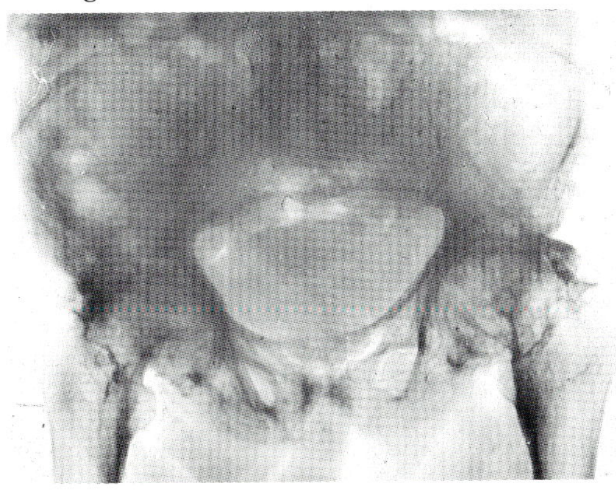

159 Paget's disease – osteolysis in skull

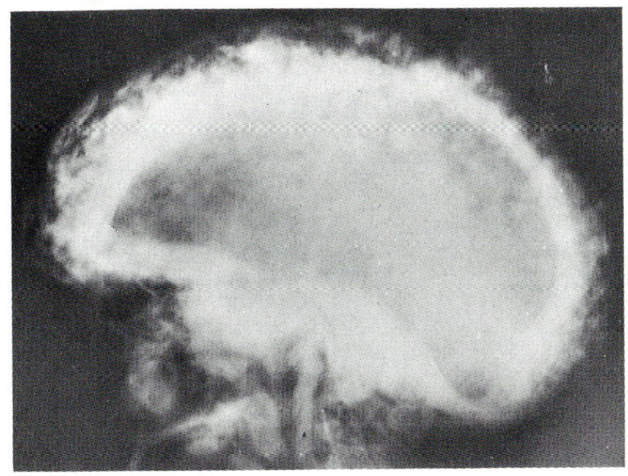

160 Paget's disease involving whole skeleton

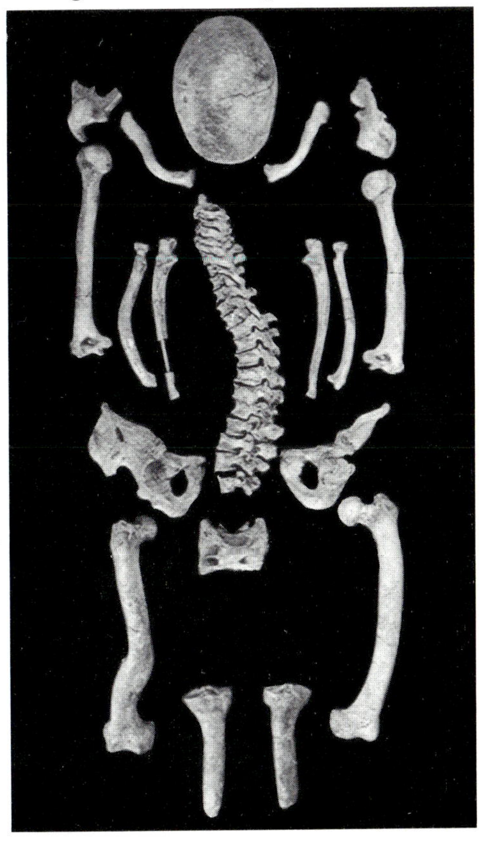

An osteosarcoma arising in the lower end of a femur thickened by Paget's disease (**161**). The incidence of malignant neoplasms of bone is increased twenty-fold in this disease. Most are osteosarcomas (60 per cent) followed by fibrosarcomas (20 per cent) and more rarely chondrosarcomas or giant cell tumours.

A myelogram shows signs of cord compression due to Paget's disease of the spine (**162**). A biopsy taken from the site of the block revealed osteosarcoma complicating Paget's disease of bone (**163** *demineralised section H&E × 350*). Note the pleomorphic hyperchromatic malignant cells and the mosaic pattern of the cement lines. Neoplasms complicating Paget's disease are more malignant than those occurring in its absence and the patient seldom survives long.

Biochemical values in Paget's disease of bone include normocalcaemia, hypercalcaemia (when complicated by fracture and bed rest or hyperparathyroidism) and rarely, hypocalcaemia when complicated by osteomalacia in the very old.

The alkaline phosphatase is often grossly increased, occasionally forty-fold, and acid phosphatase is also raised (but carcinoma of the prostate, which would also raise acid phosphatase, can coexist in the elderly male).

Skull changes can be so gross as to produce a corrugated skull (St Francis' sign, **164**).

161 Osteosarcoma complicating Paget's disease

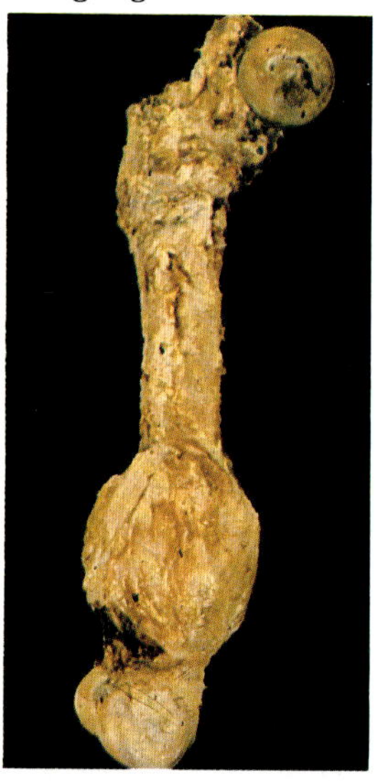

162 Paget's disease – cord compression

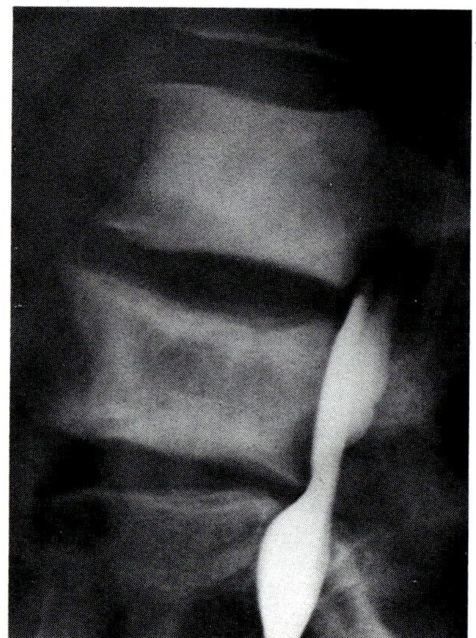

163 Osteosarcoma complicating Paget's disease

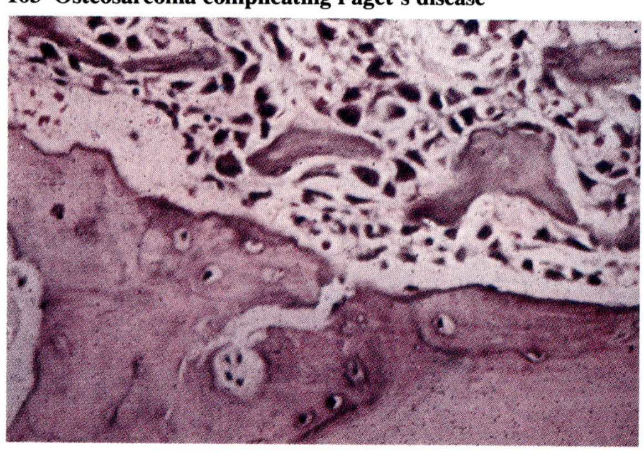

164 Corrugated skull

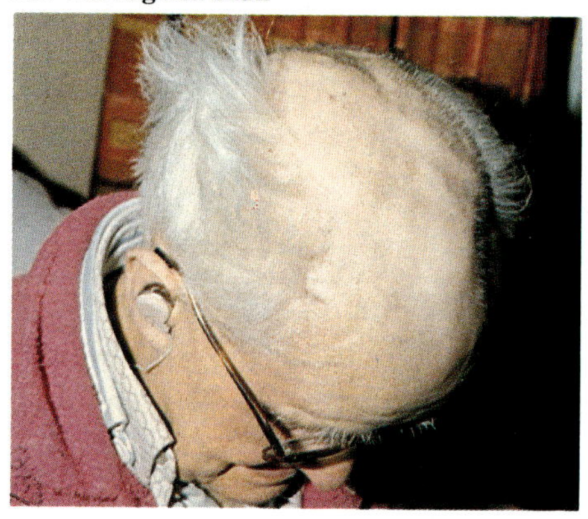

e. Renal osteodystrophy

Chronic renal failure is usually accompanied by bone disease. Some of the aetiological factors are shown in **24** on page 17. The bone lesions, which include osteomalacia, osteitis fibrosa due to secondary hyperparathyroidism, osteosclerosis and osteoporosis, are referred to as renal osteodystrophy. With the introduction of intermittent haemodialysis and therefore prolongation of life, bone disease constitutes a major problem in chronic renal failure. In the child there may be dwarfism, as in this 16 year old boy who is 1.37 m tall (**165**).

The parathyroid glands are enlarged by hyperplasia in 90 per cent of cases when examined post mortem. In most cases the hyperplasia is diffuse with loss of fat cells and a predominance of transitional and/or water clear cells. There is a correlation between the weight of the parathyroid glands and the severity of the osteitis fibrosa. In a few patients nodular hyperplasia in which glands weigh several grams is associated with severe bone disease.

Osteitis fibrosa due to secondary hyperparathyroidism occurs in practically all patients with renal osteodystrophy. The lesions can be superficial or deep. Osteoclastic resorption of bone with marrow fibrosis (**166** *mineralised section, Goldner's stain × 250*), and collections of multinucleated osteoclasts in the more severe cases (**167** *mineralised section, H&E × 120*).

165 Renal osteodystrophy – dwarfism

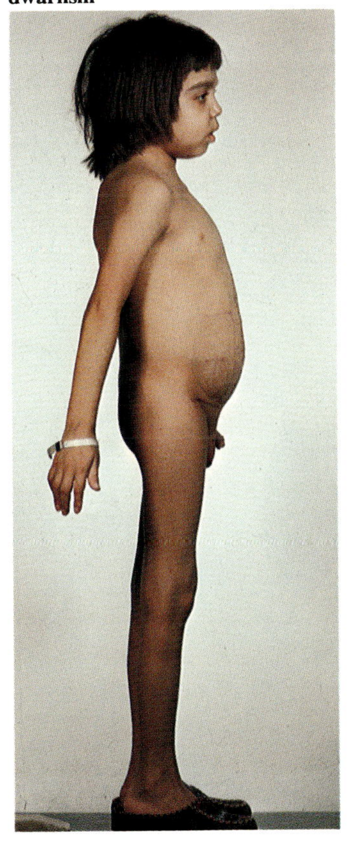

166 Osteitis fibrosa

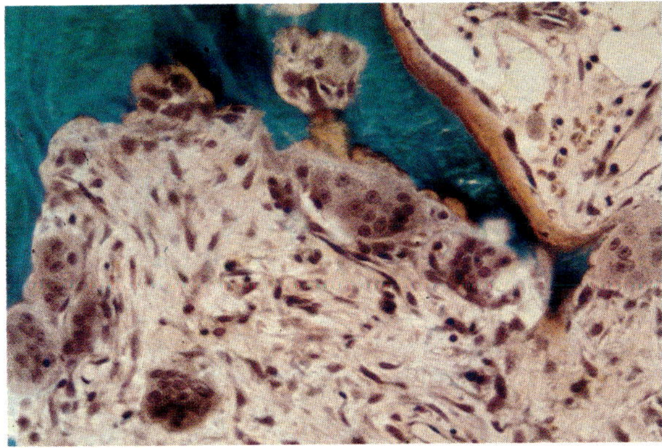

167 Osteitis fibrosa

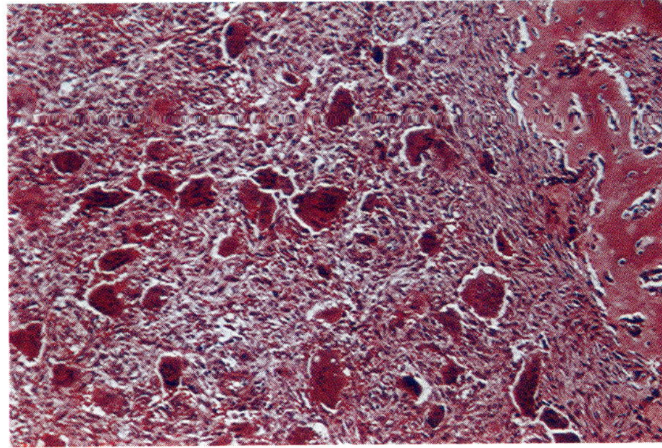

Osteomalacia seen as a large excess of osteoid five or more seams thick covering cancellous trabeculae (**168** *mineralised section, Goldner's stain* × *180*). The highest osteoid volumes are found in patients with chronic pyelonephritis.

Osteosclerosis occurs in about a third of cases. The lesion is an excess of mineralised bone with osteoid (not visible) covering most of the bone surface (**169** *demineralised section, H&E* × *60*). Fluoride retention, which occurs in chronic renal failure, may be responsible.

The alternation of sclerosis and porosis with malacia gives rise to a banded appearance of the vertebral column ('rugger jersey') (**170**).

168 Renal osteodystrophy – osteoid

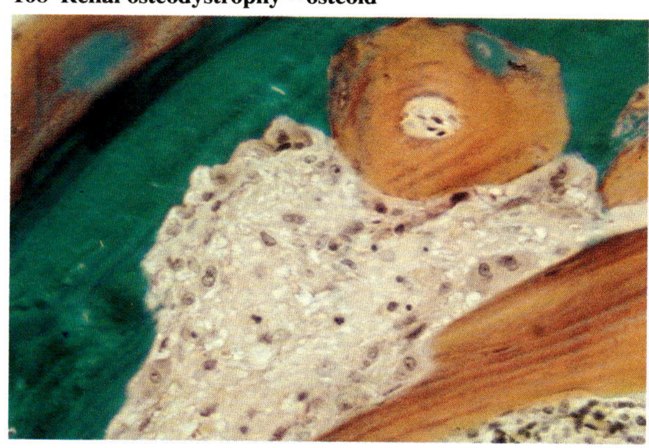

169 Osteosclerosis

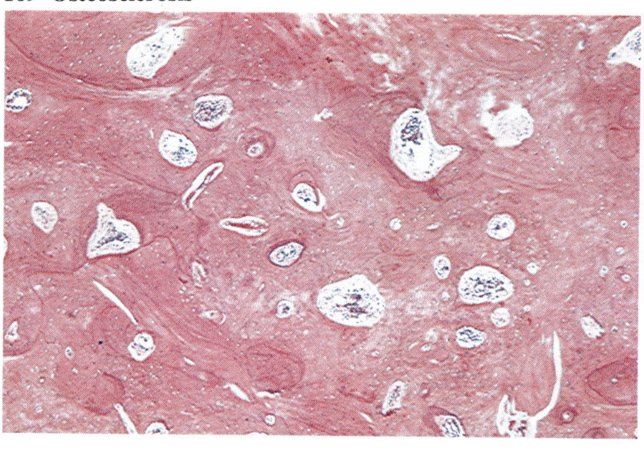

170 Sclerosis and porosis

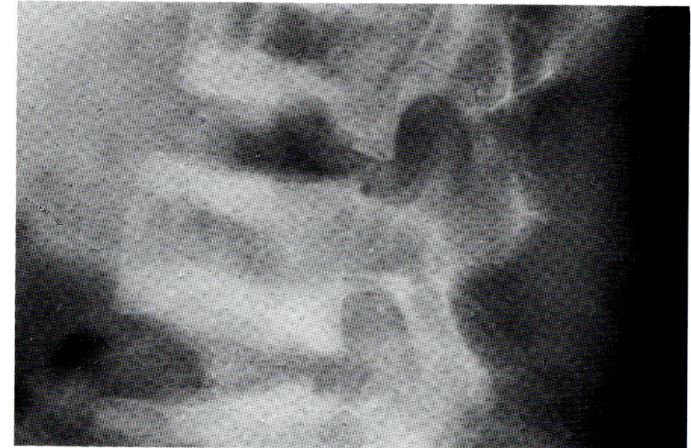

f. Hyperparathyroidism

Hyperparathyroidism may be (1) primary or (2) secondary.

1. Primary hyperparathyroidism exists when more parathyroid hormone (PTH) is produced than is needed.
2. In secondary hyperparathyroidism excess PTH is produced in response to a low ionised Ca^{++} concentration, a low Mg^{++} or a low vitamin D concentration.

The term tertiary hyperparathyroidism refers to the development of parathyroid adenomas against a background of prolonged secondary hyperparathyroidism. The differentiation histologically is fine as hyperplasia and microadenomas of four glands or one dominant adenoma may be found.

A fall in plasma calcium stimulates secretion of PTH which acts on bone to increase resorption; on the kidney to increase the excretion of phosphate and the tubular resorption of calcium; and on the gut to promote calcium absorption. The gut effect is dependent on the 1:25 dihydroxycholecalciferol concentration, the active metabolite of vitamin D. The final elaboration of vitamin D is carried out in the kidney under the control of PTH, possibly due to its effects on tubular intracellular phosphate concentration (**171**). All these effects are increased in hyperparathyroidism.

171 Control of vitamin D metabolism

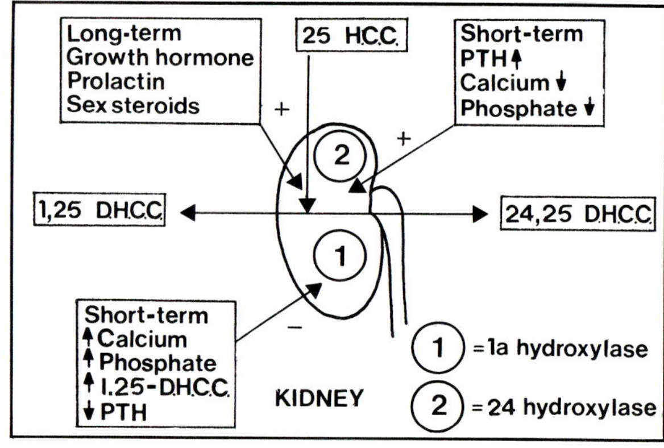

1. Primary hyperparathyroidism

Causes of primary hyperparathyroidism are:
- adenoma (or two adenomas)
- carcinoma (rare)
- hyperplasia of water clear cells or chief cells (rare)

Adenoma of one or two parathyroids accounts for more than 90 per cent of cases of primary hyperparathyroidism. Although a solitary adenoma of one of the lower parathyroids is the rule, about 6 per cent of patients have two adenomas. Adenomas are light brown in colour, soft in consistency and egg-shaped (**172**). Most adenomas weigh 1 to 5 g (normal weight of the gland 30 mg). The adenoma has a partial rim of normal parathyroid tissue which is helpful in distinguishing between adenoma and hyperplasia (**173** *H&E × 10*). Nuclear pleomorphism is commonly encountered in benign enlargements, and invasion and metastases are the most reliable indicators of malignancy.

In about 6 per cent of cases of primary hyperparathyroidism the cause is hyperplasia of all four glands (**174**). The enlargement occurs simultaneously in all glands and in the absence of a known stimulus such as renal disease or malabsorption. In long-standing hyperparathyroidism the glands may be nodular.

Primary hyperparathyroidism presents most frequently as renal calculi (**175**), the symptoms being loin pain, renal colic or haematuria. The calculi are mainly calcium phosphate and result from the high excretion of calcium. The incidence of primary hyperparathyroidism among patients with renal stones is in the order of 5 per cent, however, bone disease is rare in patients with calculi.

172 Parathyroid adenoma

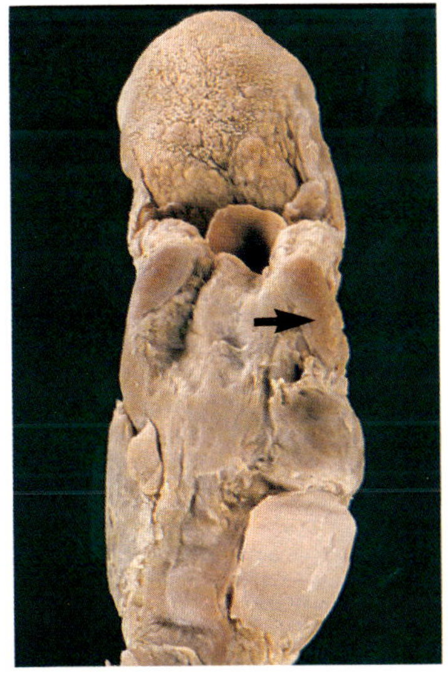

174 Parathyroid hyperplasia

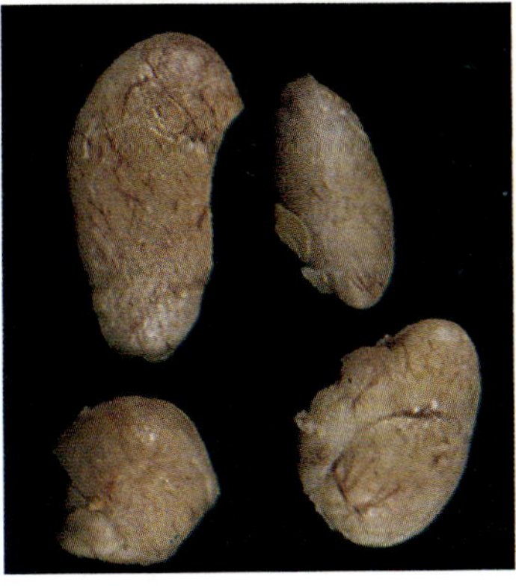

173 Adenoma with rim of normal tissue

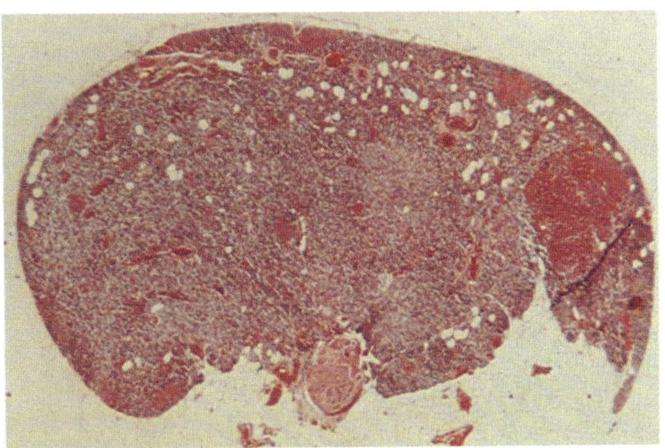

175 Hyperparathyroidism – renal calculi

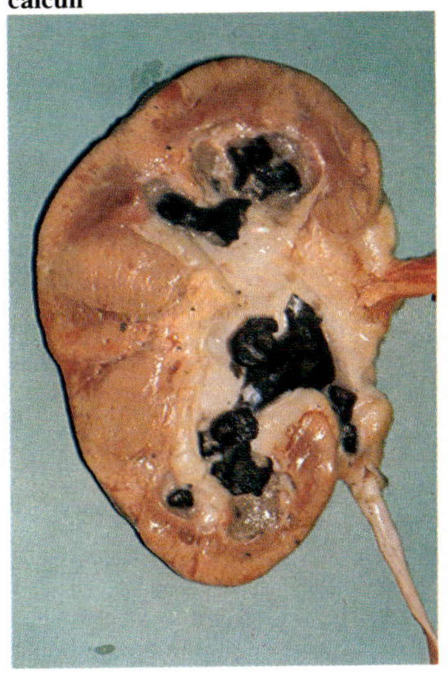

Excessive mobilisation of calcium from the bones occurs in both primary and secondary hyperparathyroidism and results in metastatic calcification, especially in the walls of arterioles, as in this section of cerebrum (**176** *H&E × 120*).

Hyperparathyroidism is the most common cause of nephrocalcinosis which is visible radiologically in about 15 per cent of cases (**177**).

Bone changes are the second most common presentation. The earliest change is demineralisation which is difficult to detect radiologically. The phalanges may show subperiosteal erosions (**178**) and even distal fracture. Loss of bone density in the skull is seen as a characteristic punctate loss of density, 'pepper pot skull'.

After long continued parathyroid activity, the bone changes of osteitis fibrosa cystica (von Recklinghausen's disease of bone) may be seen as 'brown tumours' expanding the ribs (**179**) and jaw (**180**).

176 Hyperparathyroidism – calcified vessels

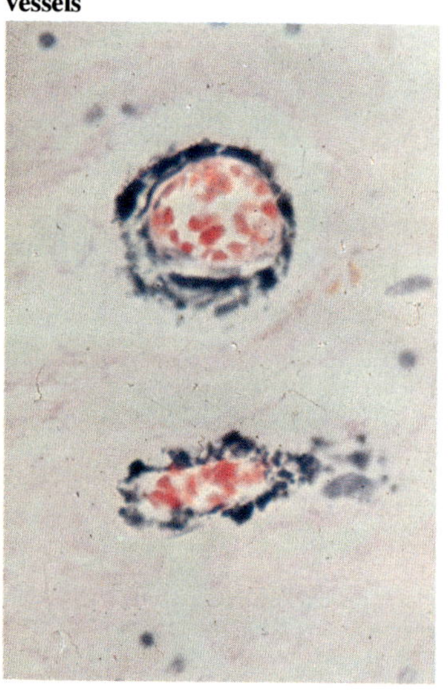

177 Nephrocalcinosis

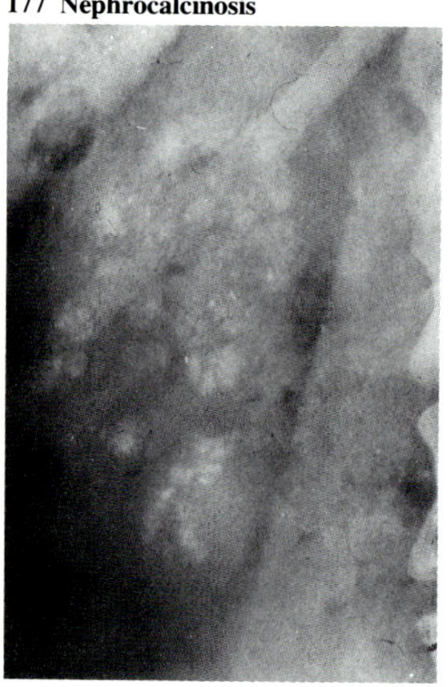

178 Hyperparathyroidism – subperiosteal erosions

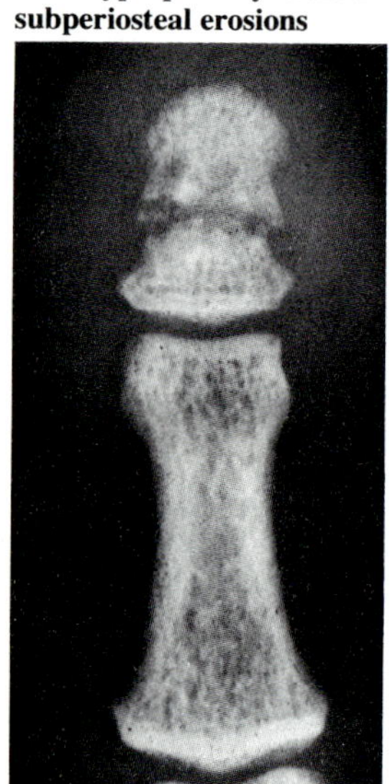

179 'Brown tumours' in rib

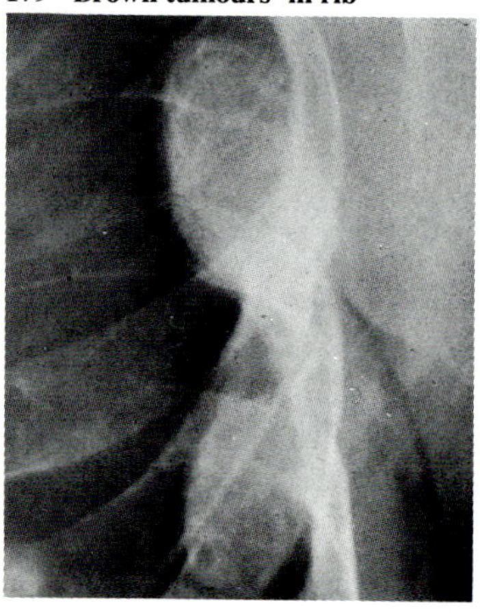

180 'Brown tumour' of jaw

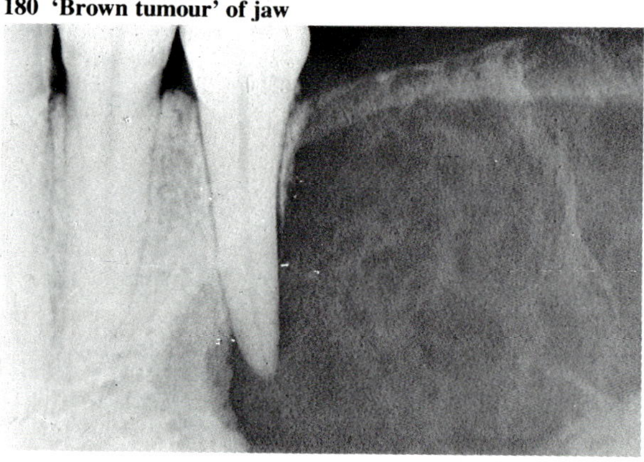

Microscopically, foci of bone destruction are seen as aggregates of giant cells in a fibrous tissue stroma (**181** *demineralised section, H&E × 350*). Skeletal deformities and pathological fractures are common. The bone lesions resolve after parathyroidectomy.

There is an increased incidence of peptic ulceration in primary hyperparathyroidism. This large duodenal ulcer was the first indication of the parathyroid lesion (**182**). A suggested pathogenesis is that a raised serum calcium causes gastrin release and consequently excess acid secretion. Other gastrointestinal symptoms include chronic constipation.

The association between primary hyperparathyroidism and pancreatitis is well recognised. In this patient with acute pancreatitis a parathyroid adenoma was found (**183**). However, hyperparathyroidism is a rare cause of this uncommon disease. The reason for the association is unknown.

Arthropathy is another recognised feature. One of the joint lesions, calcium pyrophosphate deposition in and around joints, is shown in **184**. Chondrocalcinosis, calcification of joint cartilages, is also a fairly common radiological finding in patients with long-standing hyperparathyroidism.

181 Osteitis fibrosa – bone lesion

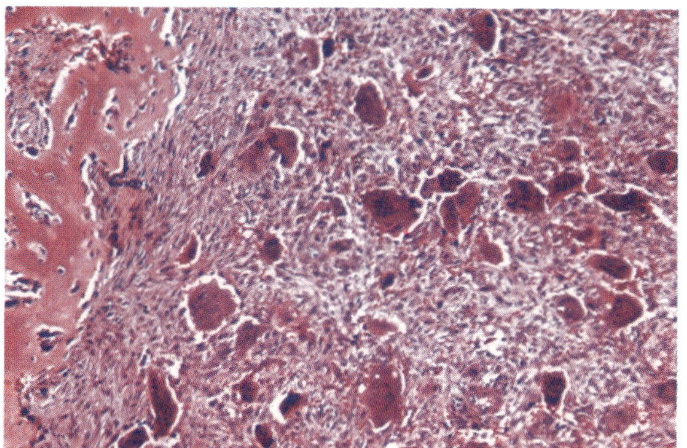

182 Peptic ulcer in hyperparathyroidism

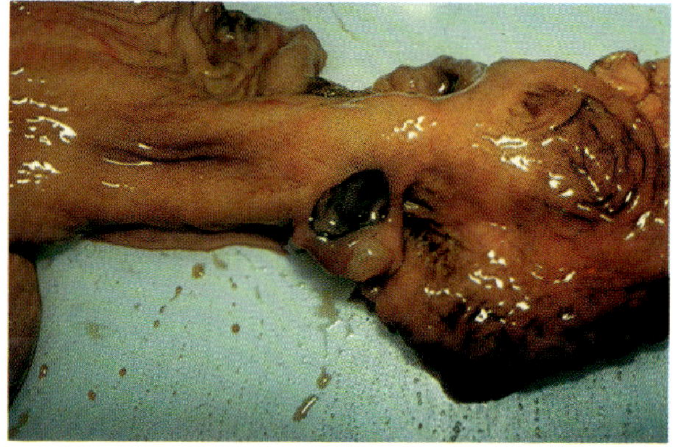

183 Acute pancreatitis

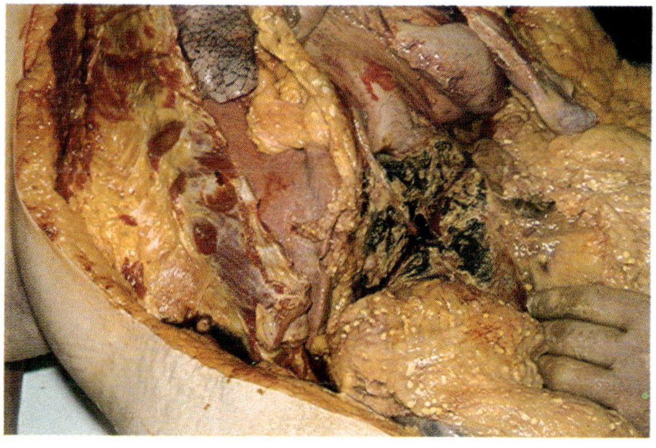

184 Chondrocalcinosis in hyperparathyroidism

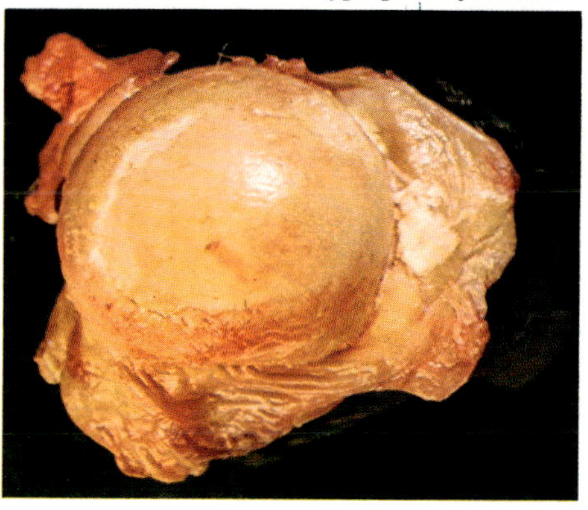

2. Secondary hyperparathyroidism

Conditions which produce a fall in the level of the plasma calcium and a compensatory parathyroid response are included under the heading of secondary hyperparathyroidism. Secondary parathyroid hyperplasia is usually associated with chronic renal failure and the malabsorption syndrome.

The common chronic renal diseases complicated by hyperparathyroidism and bone lesions (renal osteodystrophy) are polycystic kidneys, chronic pyelonephritis, chronic glomerulonephritis and hydronephrosis from any cause.

g. Multiple endocrine adenomatosis

Familial hyperparathyroidism is frequently associated with adenomas of other endocrine glands – pancreas, anterior pituitary etc. In one of these so-called pluriglandular syndromes, parathyroid hyperplasia and less commonly adenomas are associated with phaeochromocytoma, medullary thyroid cancer and more rarely, Cushing's syndrome. The differential diagnosis between the varieties of hyperparathyroidism are shown in the table below.

Biochemical findings in hyperparathyroidism		
Plasma calcium	– primary and tertiary hyperparathyroidism	– raised
	– secondary hyperparathyroidism	– normal or low
Plasma phosphorus	– primary, secondary and tertiary	– low (due to malabsorption) – high (due to renal failure)
Alkaline phosphatase	– primary, secondary and tertiary	– slightly raised except in presence of bone lesions when it can be very high

h. Osteosclerosis

In osteosclerosis there is an increase in bone mineral, trabeculae are thickened but the bone may be nevertheless more fragile to sheering strains (**185**, compare with **117**).

It occurs in a variety of conditions, for example:
- renal failure, a vertebra from a young girl showing thickened trabeculae (**186**)
- fluorosis, lumbar spine of a patient living in a high fluoridinated water area with mild renal failure showing uniform density of vertebrae (**187**)
- sclerosing metastatic deposits shown on a lateral view of thoracic spine in a patient with carcinoma of the breast (**188**). A section of the bone shows a massive increase in bone mass with deposits in the marrow (**189** *demineralised section, H&E × 60*)
- a rare metabolic disease with increased density in all the bones of the skeleton, 'marble bones' or Albers-Schoenberg disease, radiograph of the hands (**190**)

185 Osteosclerosis – bone components

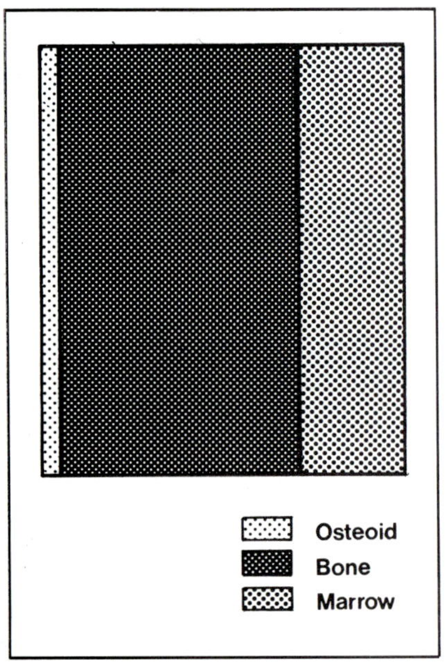

186 Osteosclerosis in renal failure

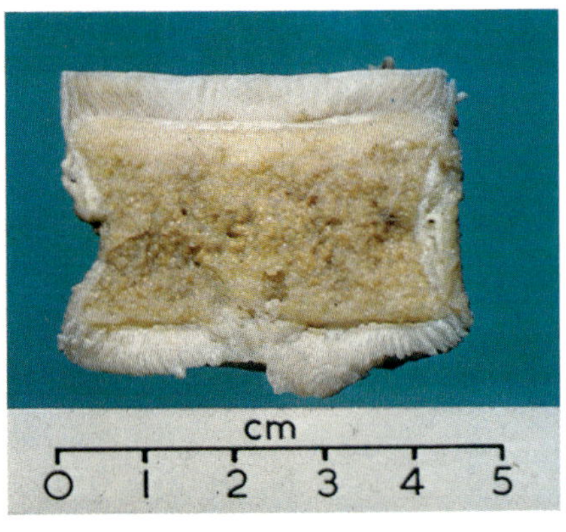

187 Osteosclerosis in fluorosis

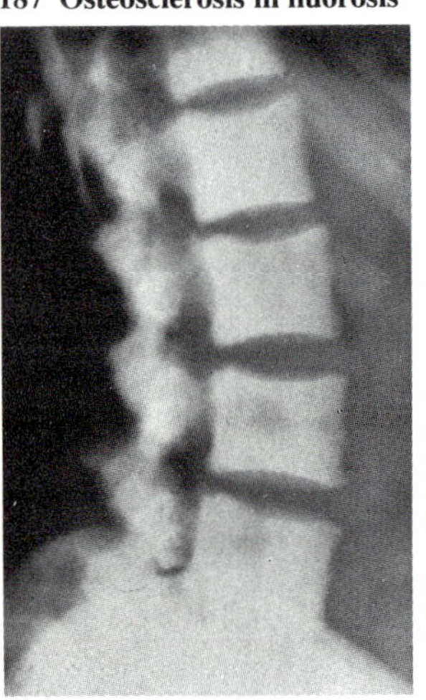

188 Sclerosing metastases in spine

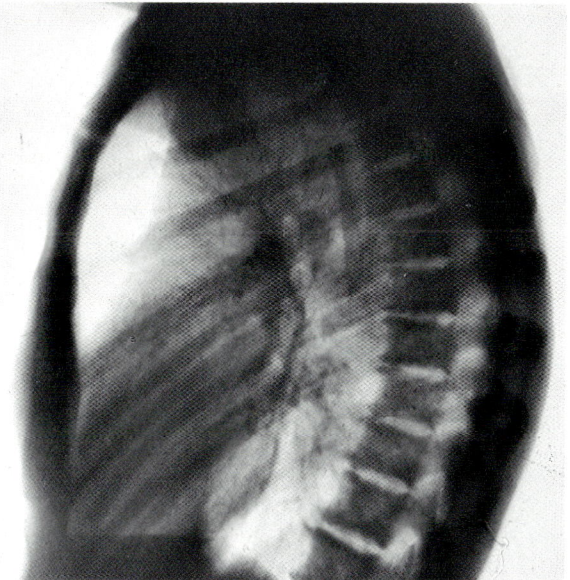

189 Sclerosing metastases

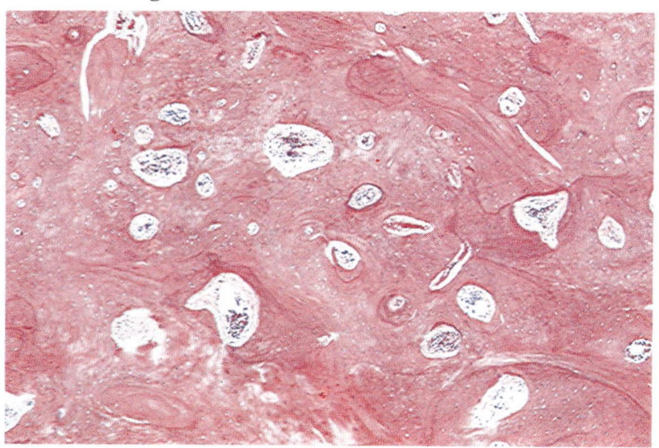

190 Albers-Schoenberg disease

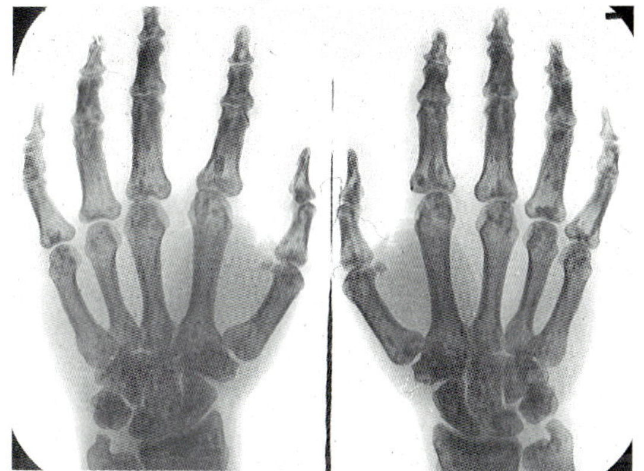

i. Isolated osteolysis

The term acro-osteolysis is used to describe adverse groups of idiopathic disorders in which lysis of the bones of the distal extremities is an outstanding feature. There are differences related to the presence or absence of genetic transmission and the association with familial renal disease. Spontaneous fracture and shortening of the phalangeal and tarsal bones are common and occasionally the mandible 'vanishes'. Radiological examination reveals resorption of the terminal phalanges and massive lytic areas in isolated bones (**191** and **192**). Pathological examination reveals that small thick-walled blood vessels have replaced the central portion of the lytic areas. The vessels were separated by fibrous tissue containing many small nerve fibres. Laboratory investigations are invariably normal.

191 Mandibular isolated osteolysis

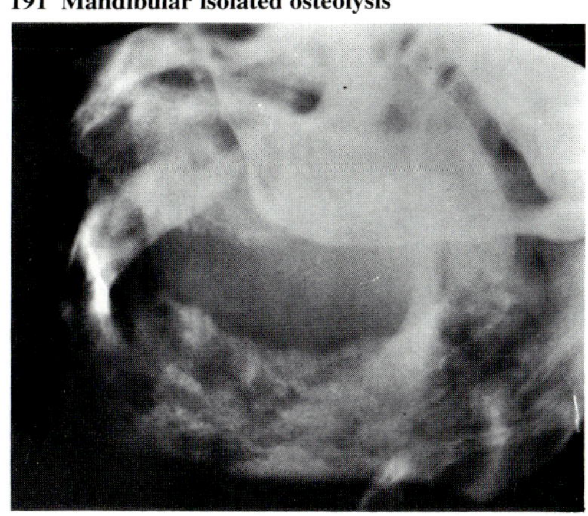

192 Mandibular isolated osteolysis

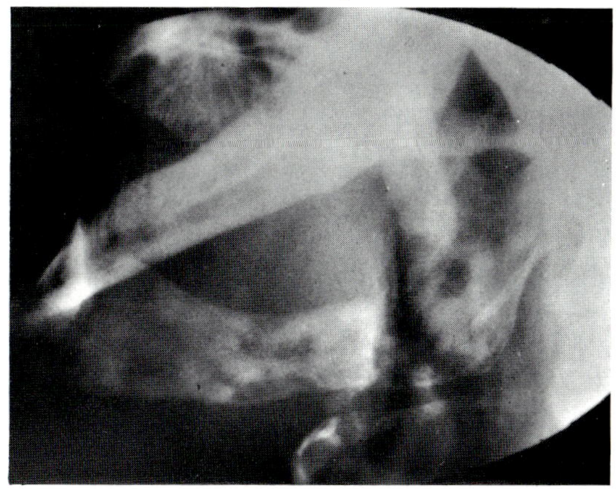

4. Tumours of bone

Tumours of bone can be classified as benign or malignant and according to the bone tissues involved.

a. Benign tumours of bone

1. Osteoma
2. Osteoid osteoma
3. Osteoblastoma
4. Haemangioma
5. Aneurysmal bone cyst
6. Simple bone cyst
7. (Reparative) granuloma of jaw
8. Osteocartilaginous exostosis
9. Chondroblastoma
10. Chondromyxoid fibroma

b. Malignant tumours of bone

1. Osteosarcoma
2. Parosteal osteosarcoma
3. Soft tissue osteosarcoma
4. Chondrosarcoma
5. Fibrosarcoma of bone
6. Giant cell tumour of bone
7. Ewing's tumour of bone
8. Adamantinoma
9. Metastatic bone tumours

c. Malignant tumours of marrow elements

1. Multiple myeloma
2. Histiocytosis
   i. Eosinophilic granuloma
   ii. Hand-Schüller-Christian disease
   iii. Letterer-Siwe disease
3. Lymphomas
4. Myeloproliferative disorders

a. Benign tumours of bone

1. Osteoma

Osteoma is a benign, slow growing neoplasm arising from the membranous bones of the face and skull (**193**). It may be composed of compact or cancellous bone and does not become malignant. Osteoma is painless but may produce a palpable tumour on the outside of the skull, cause epileptiform attacks or other symptoms by pressure inside the skull, block a nasal sinus, or produce exophthalmos.

193 Frontal sinus osteoma

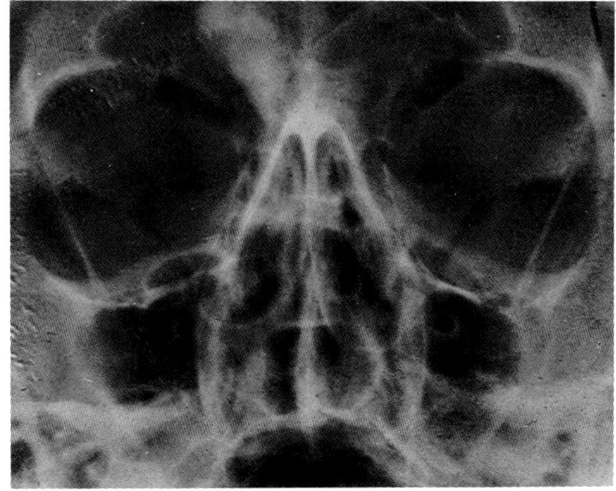

2. Osteoid osteoma

Osteoid osteoma is a benign neoplasm of osteoblasts which affects young people and shows a predilection for the long bones of the extremities. Clinically, osteoid osteoma presents with pain which may be exquisite and worse at night. A rounded focus of osteoid is present in a richly vascular connective tissue stroma (**194** *demineralised section, H&E × 50*).

The osteoid is lined by numerous plump osteoblasts and shows little or no mineralisation (**195** *demineralised section, H&E × 50*).

The typical radiological picture is of a central translucent zone surrounded by dense bone (**196**). Osteoid osteoma does not undergo involution and cure can only be effected by surgical excision.

194 Osteoid osteoma

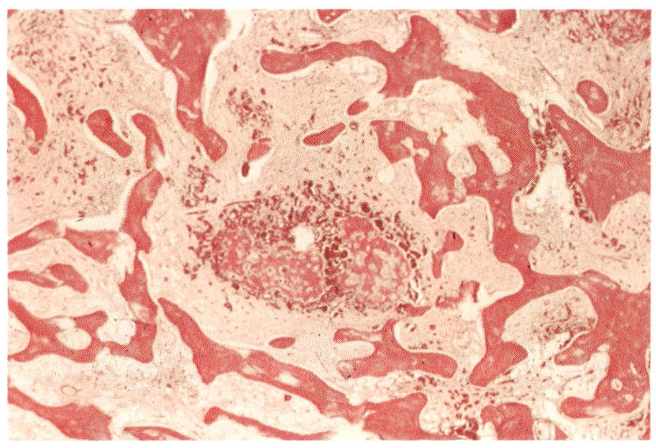

195 Osteoid osteoma – osteoblasts

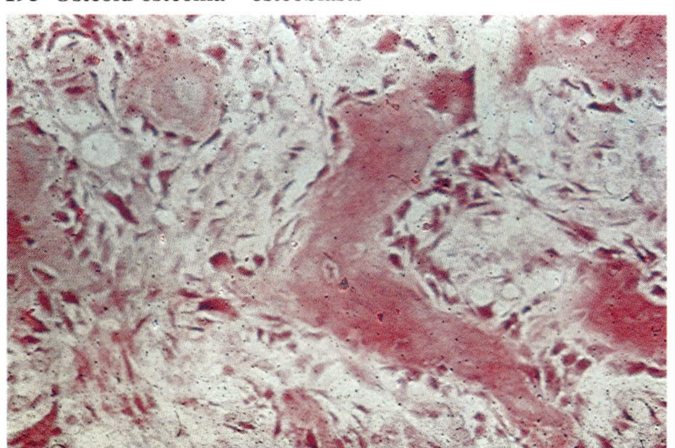

196 Osteoid osteoma – talus

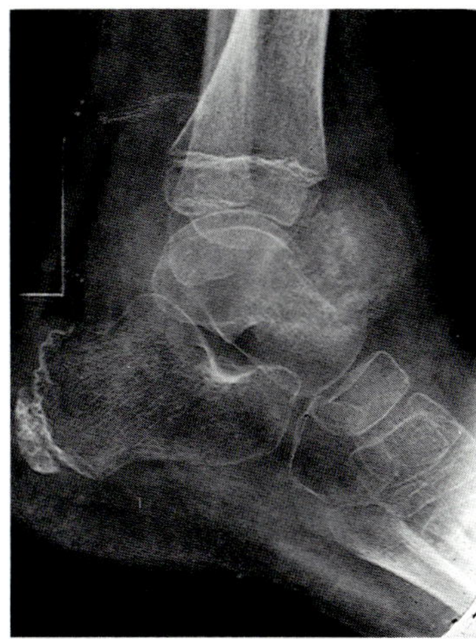

3. Osteoblastoma

Osteoblastoma is brown to red in colour, gritty in consistency and vascular enough to make haemostasis difficult. The microscopic appearances are variable, but include new bone deposition and plump osteoblasts which are uniform in appearance and lack the pleomorphism, hyperchromatism and mitotic activity seen in osteosarcoma (**197** and **198** *demineralised sections, H&E × 150 and × 80*).

197 Osteoblastoma

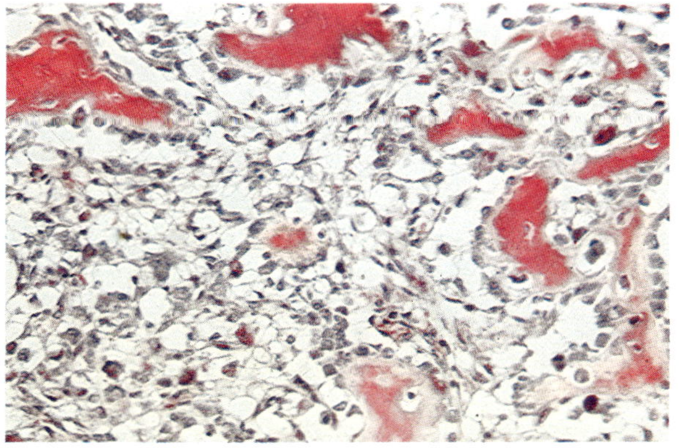

198 Osteoblastoma

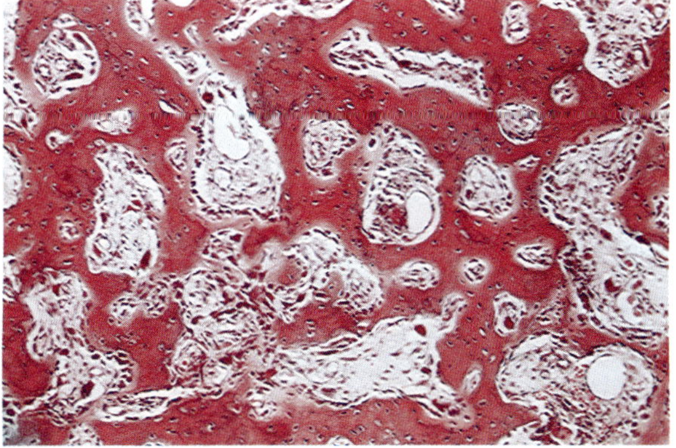

The X-ray picture is not distinctive but shows a well-circumscribed neoplasm expanding the bone and usually limited by a shell of cortical new bone. A soft tissue shadow may be present (**199**). Most patients are young and complain of pain of insidious onset which has been present for months, most commonly in the femur or tibia.

199 Osteoblastoma of maxilla

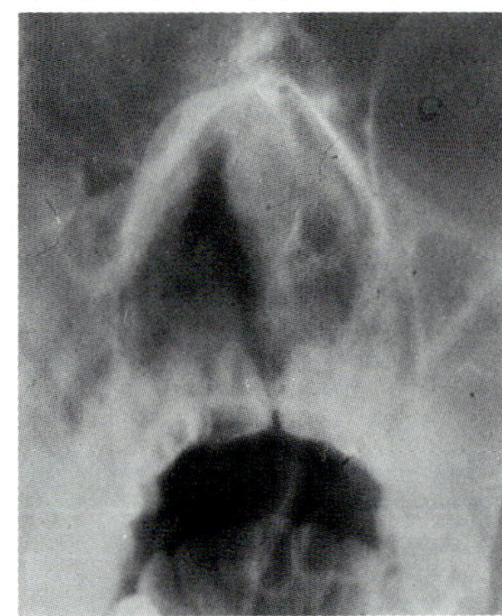

4. Haemangioma

Haemangiomas of bone are rare. Most are cavernous in type as in **200** (*demineralised section, H&E × 80*) and involve the spine, ribs and skull. Their importance lies in their ability to cause bone destruction and pathological fracture. Angiomatosis may result in massive osteolysis in adjacent bones (disappearing bone disease, **201**).

Other vascular neoplasms such as angiosarcoma are exceedingly rare.

200 Haemangioma

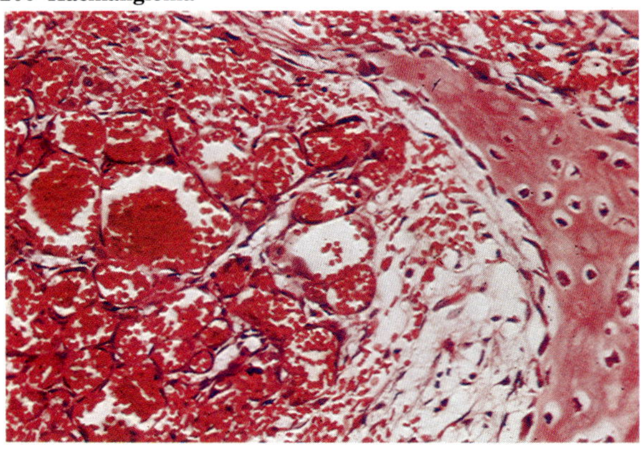

201 Osteolysis due to angiomatosis

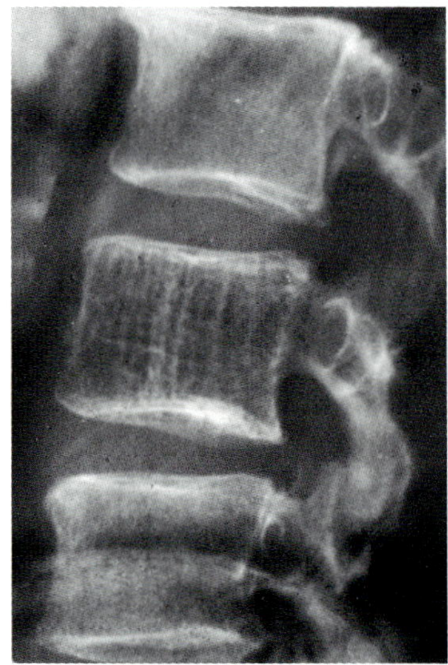

5. Aneurysmal bone cyst

Aneurysmal bone cyst is a solitary, benign, cystic lesion which expands and destroys the affected bone. The nature of the lesion is unknown but it may represent an intraosseous venous anomaly or follow trauma.

Aneurysmal bone cyst consists of vascular spaces filled with blood (**202** *demineralised section, H&E × 250*). The walls of the vascular spaces consist of vascular fibrous connective tissue containing haemosiderin laden macrophages (**203** *demineralised section, H&E × 250*). The spaces are not lined by endothelium. Macroscopically it appears as a brown blood-filled sponge.

Aneurysmal bone cyst shows central rarefaction surrounded by a thin shell of cortex. The shafts of long bones and the vertebrae are most commonly involved. The peak incidence is in the second decade of life and the patient presents with localised pain, tenderness, limitation of movement and swelling.

202 **Aneurysmal bone cyst**

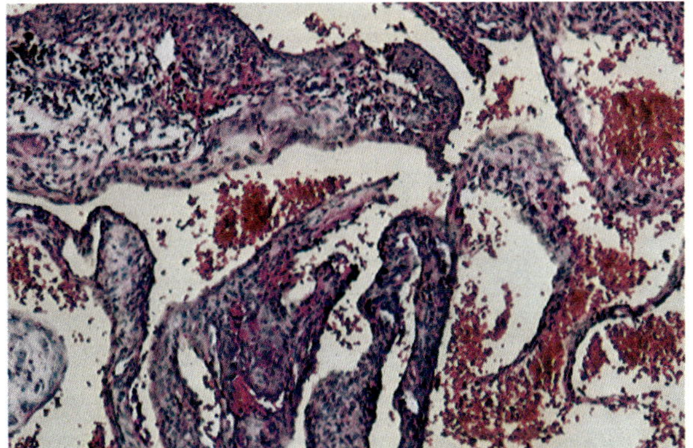

203 **Aneurysmal bone cyst**

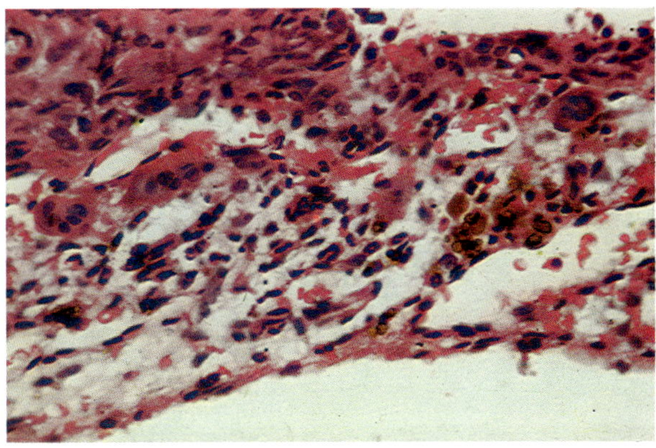

6. Simple bone cyst

Simple bone cyst (unicameral or solitary bone cyst) occurs most frequently in young males and is most commonly seen at the upper end of the humerus. The cyst contains clear fluid or, if pathological fracture occurs, organised blood clot. It is lined by fibrous tissue containing multinucleated giant cells, macrophages and osteoid. It is centrally situated and may cause atrophy and thinning of the cortex but it seldom expands the bone. The cyst shown here in the head of the humerus (**204**) is well demarcated and may, because of the presence of bony ridges, appear loculated. At first the cyst is in contact with the epiphyseal plate, but as the bone grows it appears to migrate in the metaphysis away from the plate.

204 **Simple bone cyst**

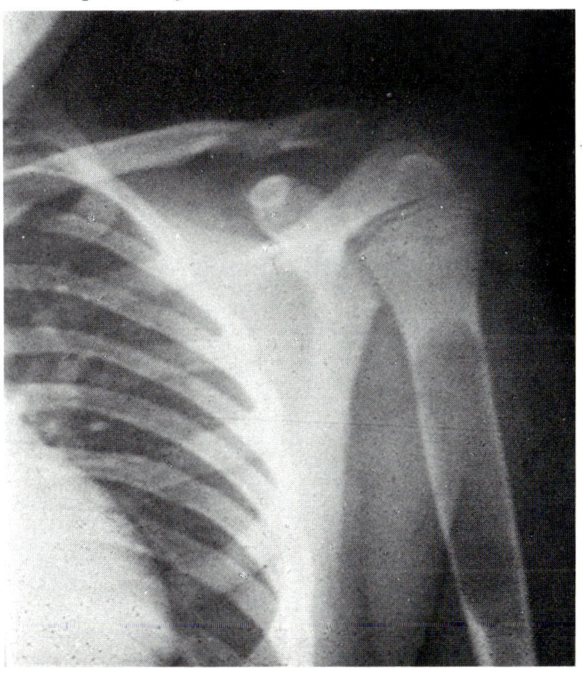

7. (Reparative) granuloma of jaw

(Reparative) granuloma (**205** *H&E × 250*) is a florid giant cell reaction in the cancellous bone of the jaw. Its causation is uncertain. Most giant cell lesions of the jaw, although resembling giant cell tumours, are non-neoplastic (reparative) granulomas.

205 **(Reparative) granuloma of jaw**

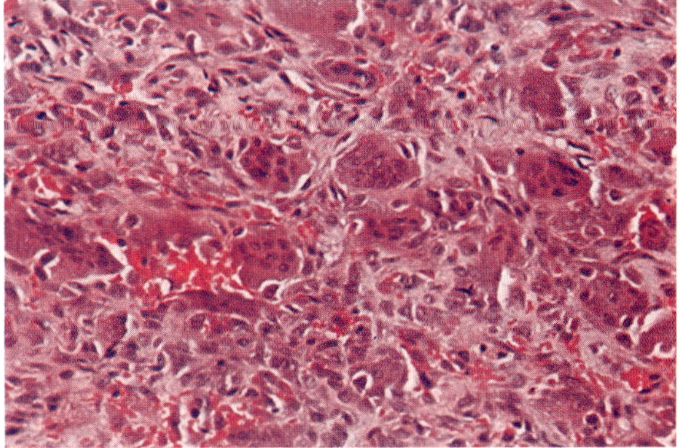

8. Osteocartilaginous exostosis

The lesion consists of a mass of trabecular bone attached to the normal bone and covered by a layer of cartilage which may be incomplete. The lesion is either broad based as in **206**, or pedunculated.

A demineralised section of the exostosis shows cartilage covering trabeculated bone (**207** *H&E × 80*).

Osteocartilaginous exostoses are thought to develop from the periosteum or from the periphery of an epiphyseal cartilaginous plate.

Exostoses are most common at the lower end of the femur and the upper end of the tibia and humerus. See **208** for distribution.

Malignant transformation of a solitary exostosis to chondrosarcoma is rare but should be suspected if there is resumption of growth in adult life or if a soft tissue shadow develops.

Hereditary multiple exostoses are inherited as an autosomal dominant. There is a greatly increased risk of malignant change.

206 Osteocartilaginous exostosis

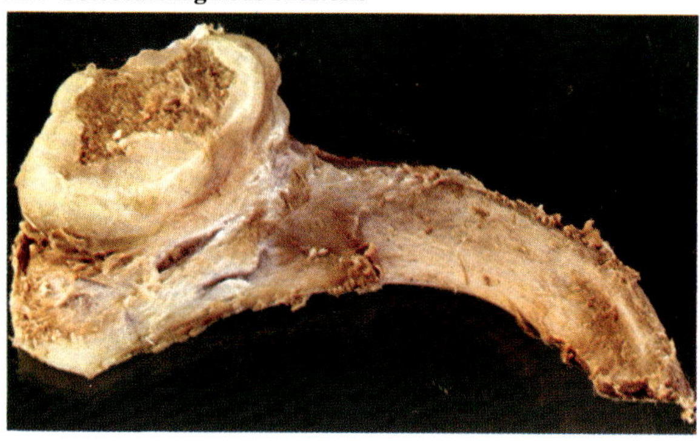

207 Osteocartilaginous exostosis

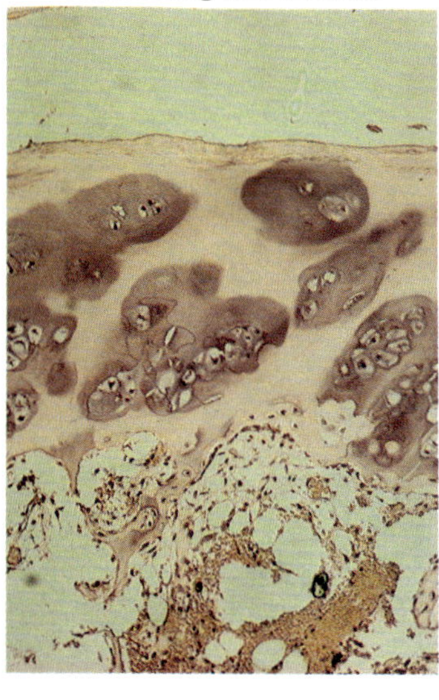

208 Osteocartilaginous exostosis – distribution

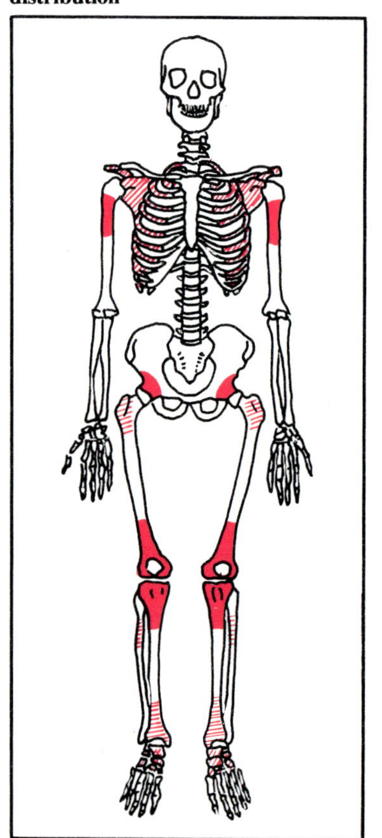

9. Chondroblastoma

A rare benign neoplasm of young people that arises in the epiphyses of a long bone adjacent to the epiphyseal cartilage plate.

Chondroblastoma, as the name indicates, is composed mainly of polygonal chondroblast-like cells (**209** *demineralised section, H&E × 200*). Other elements are giant cells and small amounts of cartilaginous matrix. Focal calcification is common. Chondroblastoma merges with chondromyxoid fibroma (see below) and both may recur after curettage.

209 Chondroblastoma

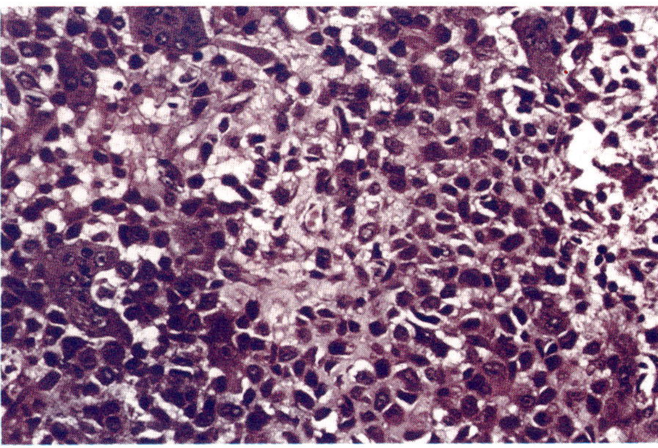

10. Chondromyxoid fibroma

Chondromyxoid fibroma is a rare benign lesion that occurs most frequently in young adults. Any tubular bone may be involved but the most common site is around the knee joint in the metaphysis of the femur and tibia.

The neoplasm arises in the medullary cavity and erodes the cortex to give a sharply outlined radiolucent area with a thin sclerotic border (**210**).

Histologically, the lesion consists of lobules of chondromyxoid tissue separated by fibrous connective tissue. Some areas may differentiate into cartilage. Scattered multinucleated giant cells and large pleomorphic cells may be present. Malignant change is rare, but failure to remove the lesion completely results in a high recurrence rate (**211** *demineralised section, H&E × 120*).

210 Chondromyxoid fibroma

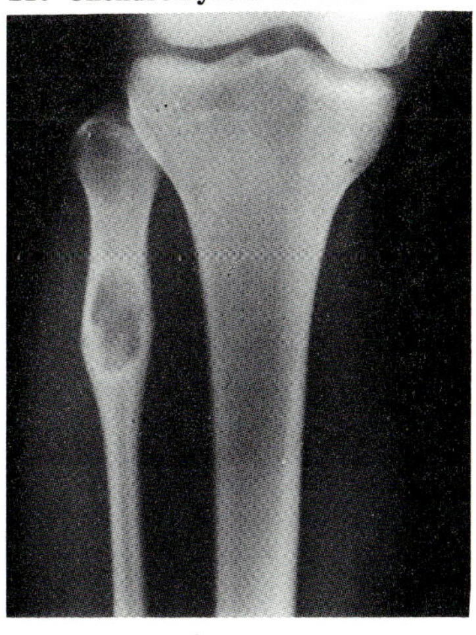

211 Chondromyxoid fibroma

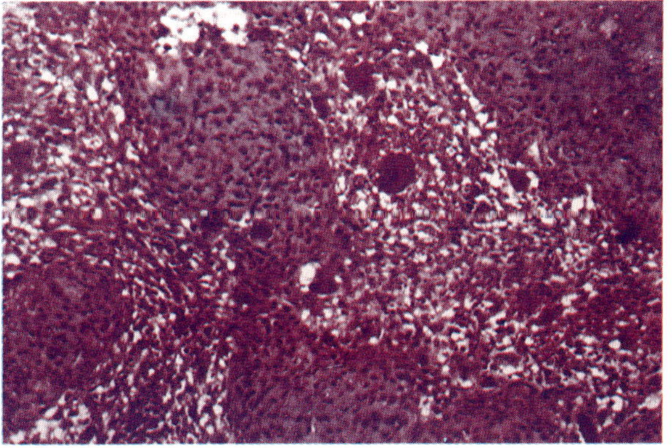

b. Malignant tumours of bone

1. Osteosarcoma

Osteosarcoma is a sarcoma in which osteoid and bone are formed by a malignant proliferation of primitive bone-forming mesenchyme. It is the commonest primary malignant neoplasm of bone. See **212** for the skeletal distribution. Most patients are males aged 10 to 20 years. A second small peak incidence occurs late in life because of an association with Paget's disease of bone. Pain, swelling and a limp are common early symptoms.

Osteosarcoma arising from the metaphysis of the lower end of the femur. A vascular mass expands the bone and grows into the soft tissues (**213**). The cut surface reveals a variety of appearances; bone, osteoid, cartilage, haemorrhage and necrosis (**214**). Spread has occurred along the medullary cavity.

A soft tissue and bony mass perforating the cortex and raising the periosteum to produce a wedge of ossification (Codman's triangle) and vertical spicules of bone. A lesion is always seen on X-ray and the presence of a soft tissue mass is characteristic of osteosarcoma (**215**).

The presence of neoplastic osteoid (pink material) and a sarcomatous stroma is essential for the diagnosis of osteosarcoma. The cells are malignant mesenchymal cells (**216** *demineralised section, H&E × 250*).

Blood spread leads to pulmonary metastases. Two small metastases, one in the upper lobe and the other in the lower lobe of the left lung are shown in **217**.

Micrometastases are often present in the lungs early in the disease. Some of the malignant osteoid shown in **218** (*demineralised section, H&E × 80*) is mineralised. The prognosis, once deplorable with a 5 year survival rate of 15 per cent, is now much improved due to the use of adjuvant chemotherapy.

212 Osteosarcoma – distribution

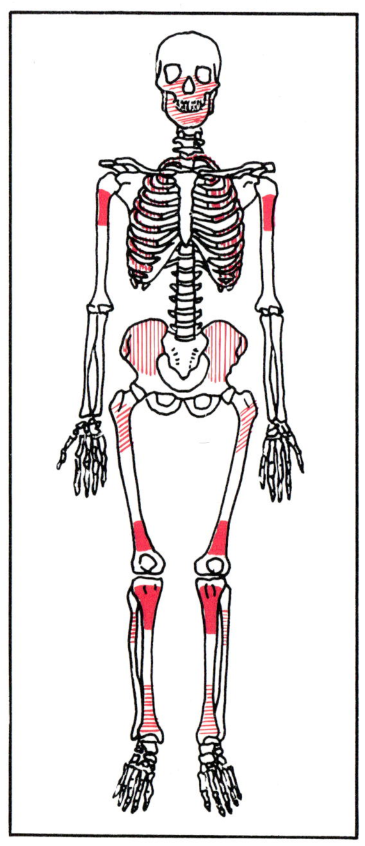

213 Osteosarcoma of femur

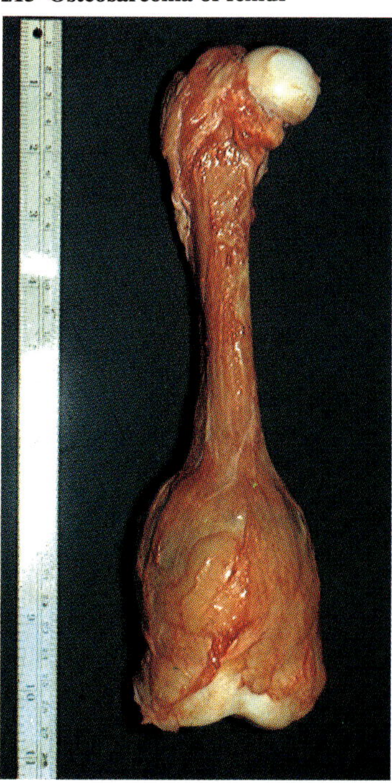

214 Osteosarcoma of femur

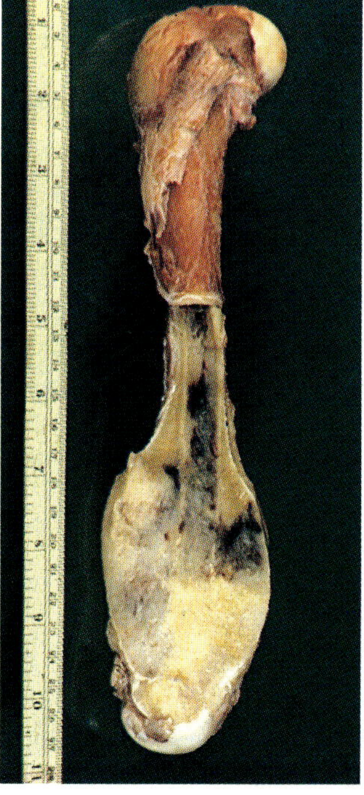

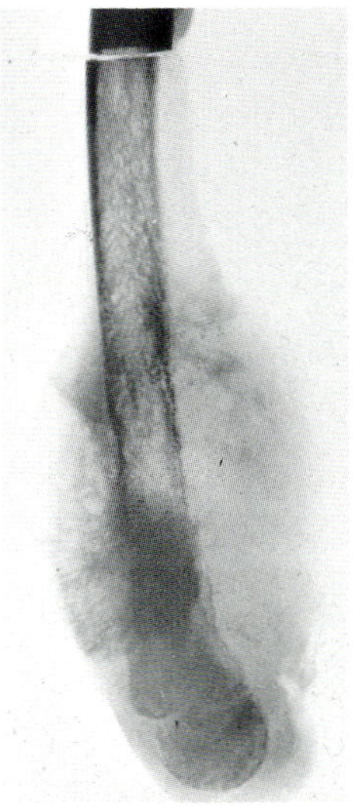

215 Osteosarcoma of femur

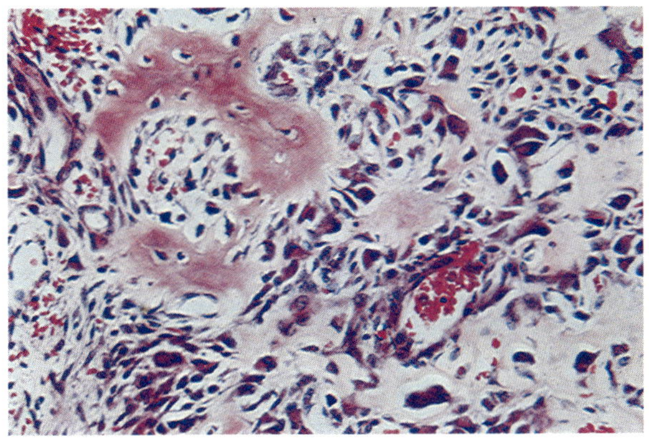

216 Osteosarcoma

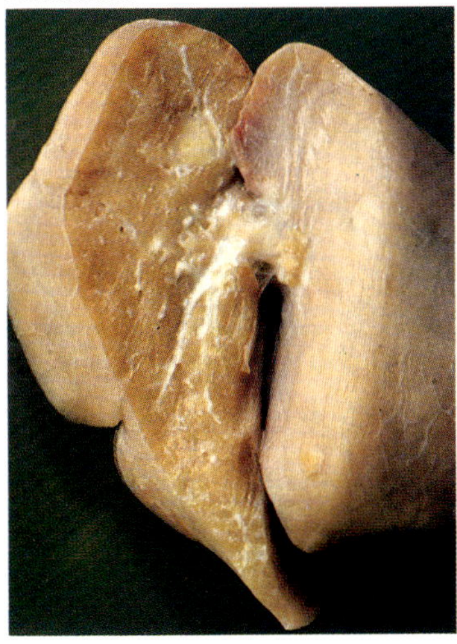

217 Osteosarcoma – pulmonary metastases

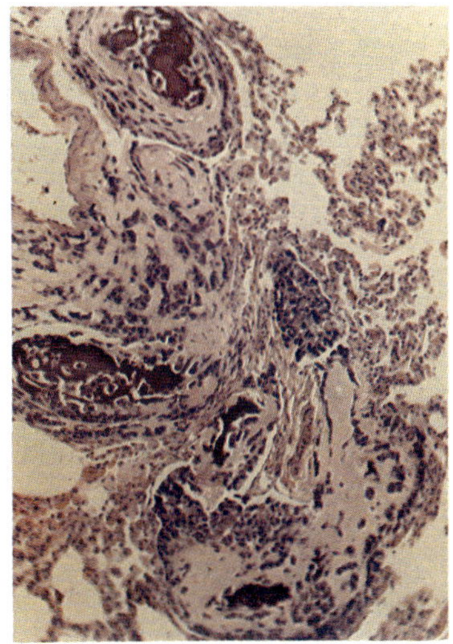

218 Osteosarcoma – micrometastases in lung

The vascularity of osteosarcoma, as seen in this specimen from the lower end of the femur (**219**), should be emphasised. Vascular spaces may be lined by malignant cells thereby permitting their ready dissemination (**220** *H&E × 250*).

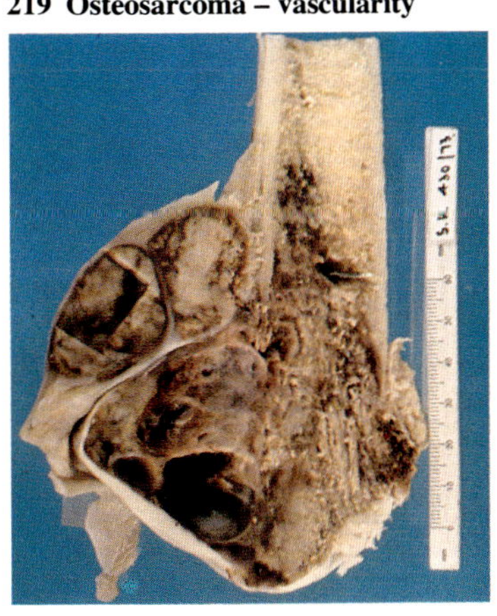

219 Osteosarcoma – vascularity

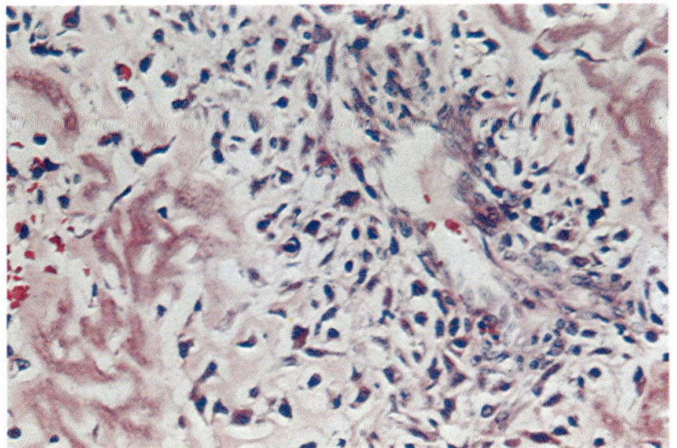

220 Osteosarcoma – vascular space

While the hallmark of osteosarcoma is the production of malignant osteoid and bone, other types of malignant tissue, especially chondrosarcoma may be present. A biopsy may consist entirely of malignant cartilage so that problems of diagnosis arise (**221** *H&E × 200*).

About half the osteosarcomas occurring over the age of 40 are associated with Paget's disease of bone. The commonest sites are the femur and humerus (**222**). Rarely, several bones may be involved by independent primary sarcomas. In these cases the prognosis is extremely poor.

221 Osteosarcoma – malignant cartilage

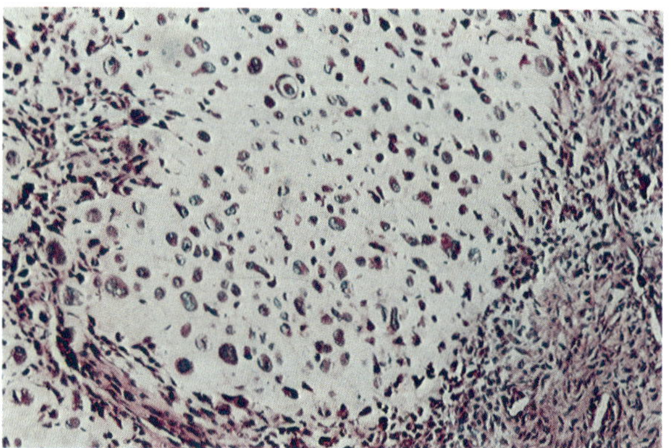

222 Osteosarcoma in Paget's disease

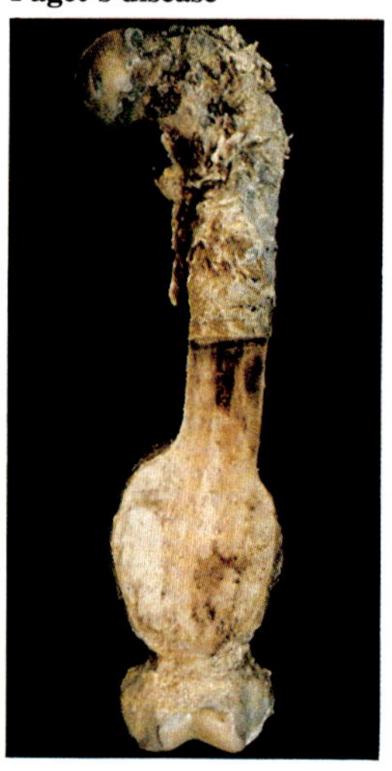

2. Parosteal osteosarcoma

Parosteal or juxtacortical osteosarcoma is a variant of osteosarcoma which develops on the surface of a bone and is closely related to the periosteum. It is a relatively rare, slow growing neoplasm compared with the more common intraosseous osteosarcoma.

The typical parosteal osteosarcoma is a lobulated mass attached by a broad base to the periosteum. With continued growth the neoplasm tends to surround the involved bone and invade the cortex. It consists mainly of bone but softer areas of cartilage and fibrous tissue are invariably present. This hard, painless mass was excised from a child (**223** *demineralised section, H&E*).

The neoplasm is seen as a sharply defined radiopaque shadow of varying density much of which is separated from the cortex by a radiolucent zone representing connective tissue (**224**).

223 Parosteal osteosarcoma

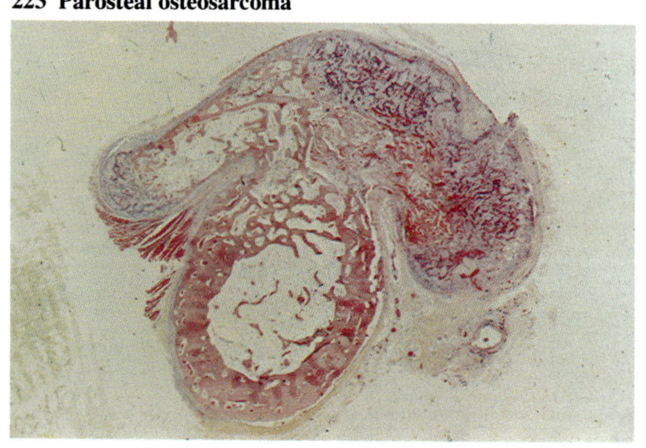

224 Parosteal osteosarcoma

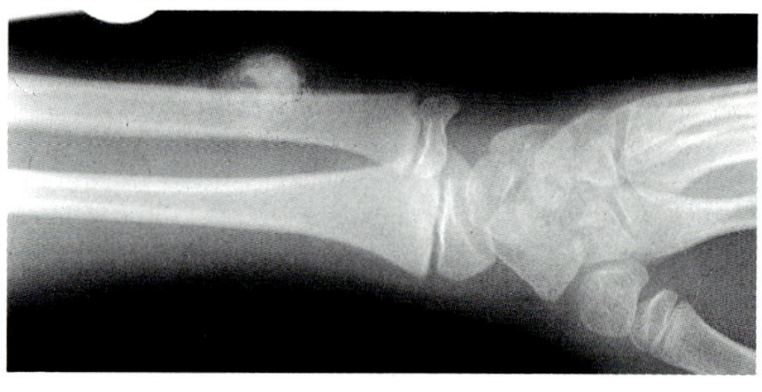

Microscopy shows varying amounts of malignant osteoid, fibrous and cartilaginous tissue surrounding trabeculae of bone (**225** and **226** *demineralised sections, H&E × 200*). Parosteal osteosarcoma has a less malignant appearance and a better prognosis than conventional osteosarcoma. About 80 per cent of patients survive 5 years but recurrence and metastases may occur later than this.

225 Parosteal osteosarcoma

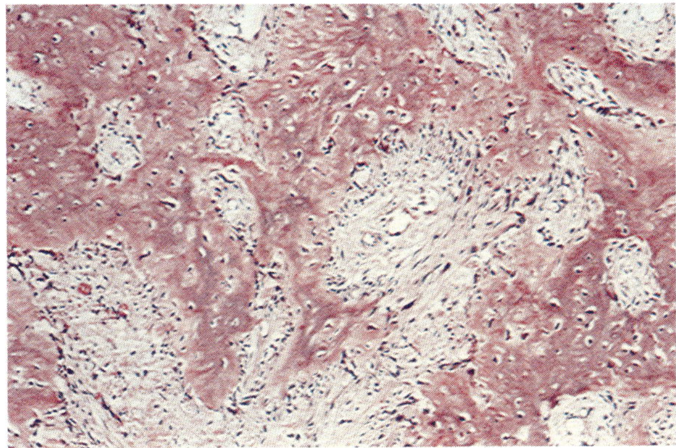

226 Parosteal osteosarcoma

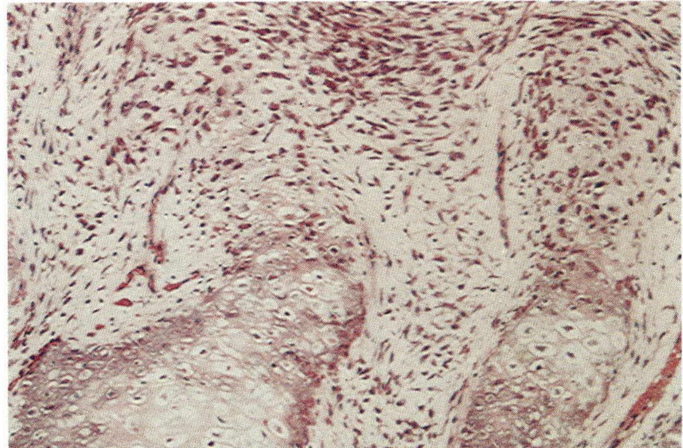

3. Soft tissue osteosarcoma

The occurrence of osteosarcoma outside the skeleton is rare. Generally, as in skeletal osteosarcoma, the lower extremities are most commonly involved. Nevertheless, this neoplasm is also found in such unusual sites as female breast, penis and pulmonary artery.

An osteosarcoma arising from and invading the soft tissues behind the knee joint (**227**). Some soft tissue osteosarcomas arise de novo from mesenchymal cells; others are believed to have arisen in previously benign neoplasms, in myositis ossificans, or following radiation. Sometimes a history of trauma is obtained but this is probably coincidental.

Radiologically, soft tissue swelling and patchy density are visible (**228**). The bones are not involved.

227 Soft tissue osteosarcoma

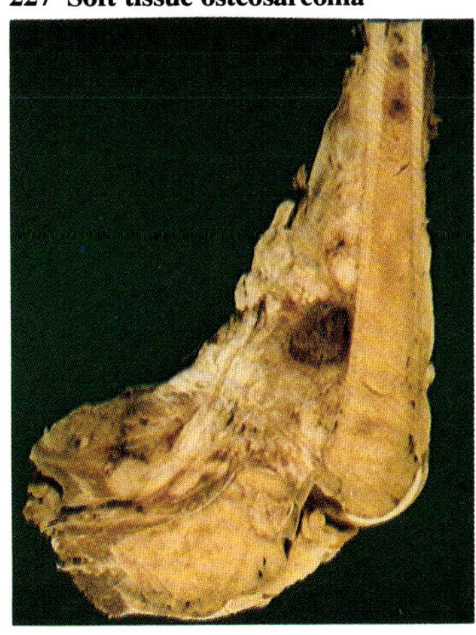

228 Soft tissue osteosarcoma

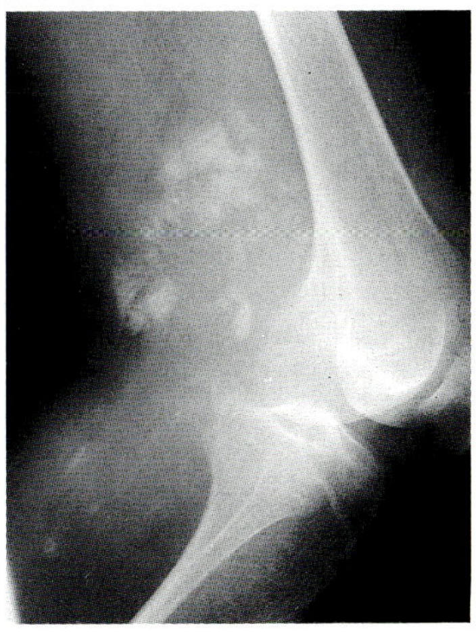

Microscopy shows an irregular meshwork of bone, osteoid and pleomorphic, hyperchromatic, neoplastic cells (**229** *demineralised section, H&E × 250*). The zoning of the tissue so characteristic of myositis ossificans is absent.

Soft tissue osteosarcoma metastasis in the right lower lobe of the lung (**230**). The prognosis is extremely poor.

229 Soft tissue osteosarcoma

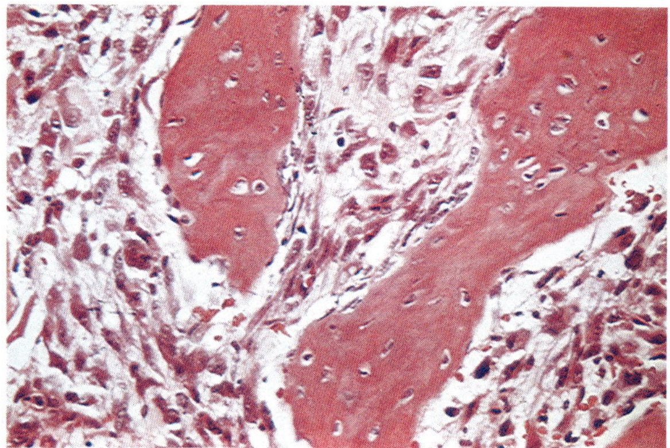

230 Soft tissue osteosarcoma – pulmonary metastasis

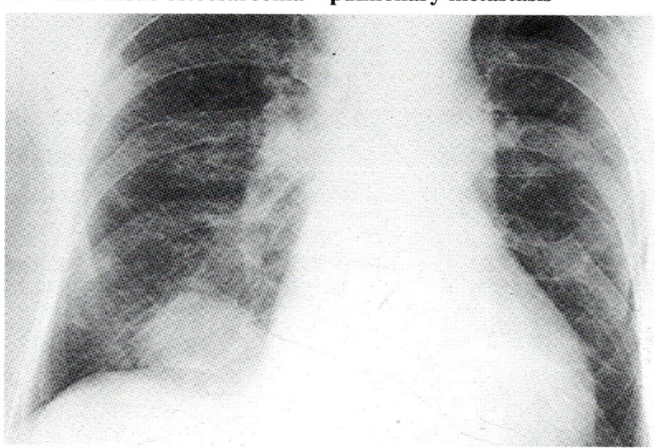

4. Chondrosarcoma

Chondrosarcomas are malignant bone neoplasms composed of cartilage and cartilaginous matrix. They are less common than osteosarcomas but both are found more frequently in males than in females. They tend to occur later than osteosarcomas, most arising over the age of 30 years. The common sites are shown in **231**. Pain and swelling are the usual presenting complaints. Chondrosarcomas can be classified as peripheral and central.

A typical peripheral chondrosarcoma, a smooth-surfaced, rounded, nodular neoplasm arising from the surface of the femur (**232**). Most peripheral chondrosarcomas are large and may be heavily mineralised. A small number develop in exostoses particularly when these are multiple.

231 Chondrosarcoma – distribution

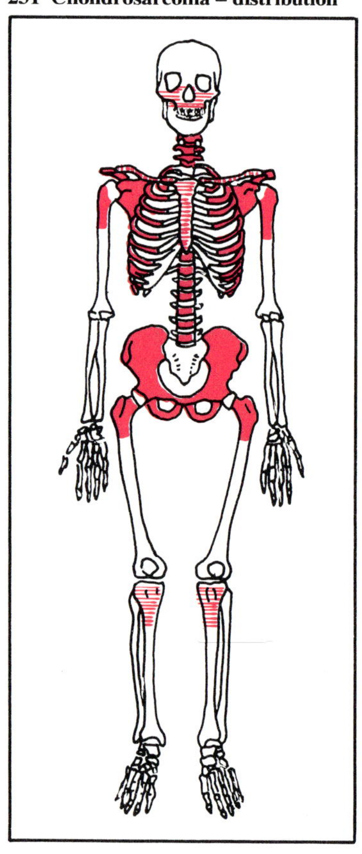

232 Chondrosarcoma of femur

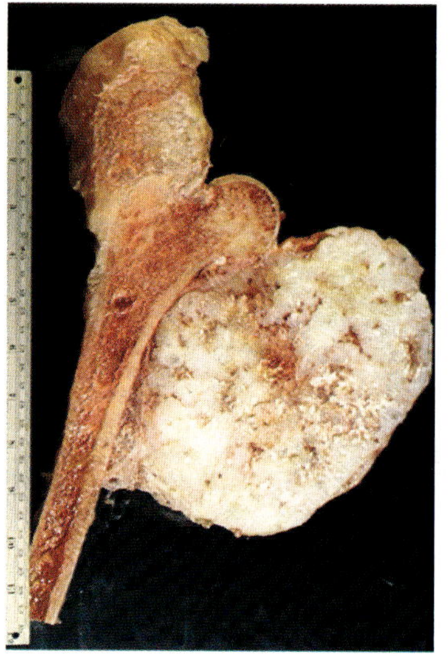

A central chondrosarcoma within the medullary cavity is expanding the humerus (**233**). The cortex is slightly thickened by subperiosteal reactive bone.

A chondrosarcoma arising from and partly destroying the innominate bone, the most common site (**234**). Chondrosarcomas may remain locally invasive for years before invading veins and metastasizing to the lungs.

An X-ray of the neoplasm shown in **234** shows destruction of the bone (**235**). The characteristic feature is an expanding lesion arising from an area of bone. The lesion is often seen as a bunch of expanding grapes faintly outlined in the periphery by calcification.

Most chondrosarcomas show areas of well-differentiated cells and therefore the microscopical differentiation between a benign and malignant cartilaginous neoplasm can be difficult. Binucleate or multinucleate cells as seen in **236** (*demineralised section, H&E × 180*) and nuclear atypia manifest as hyperchromatism, and variations in shape and size (**237** *demineralised section, H&E × 300*) indicate malignancy. Invasion of the soft tissues (on left of picture in **237**) confirms the diagnosis of chondrosarcoma.

Malignant cartilage cells readily implant if spilled into the wound during surgery. Local recurrence is the major cause of unsuccessful treatment. Although the biological behaviour of chondrosarcoma is notoriously unpredictable, the prognosis in the adult is good; 75 per cent of patients, if adequately treated, survive 5 years.

233 Central chondrosarcoma

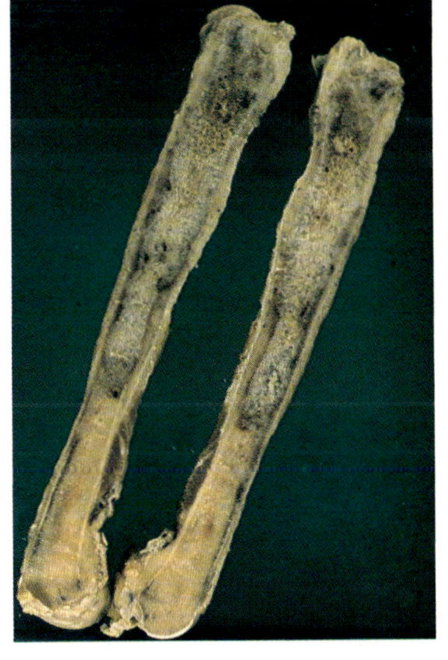

234 Chondrosarcoma of innominate bone

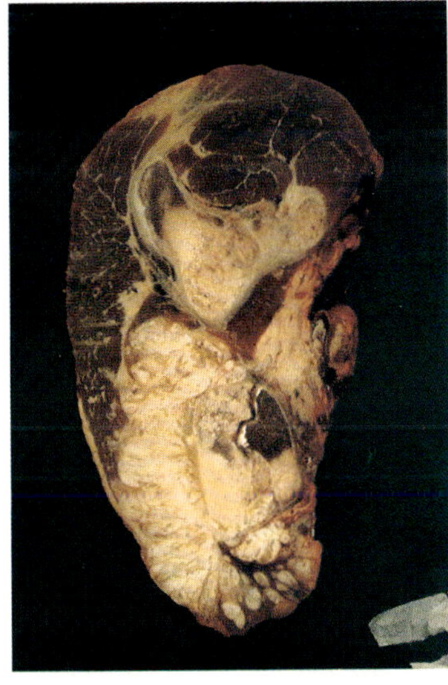

235 Chondrosarcoma of innominate bone

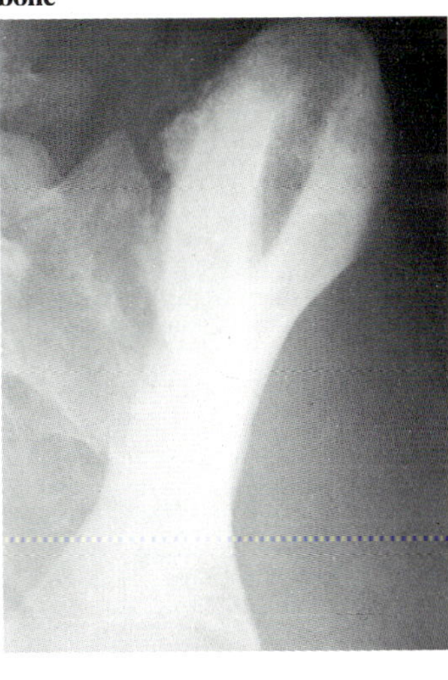

236 Chondrosarcoma – multinucleate cells

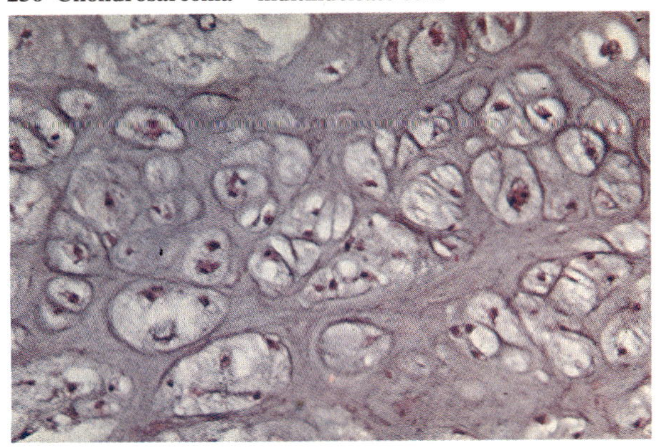

237 Chondrosarcoma – invasion of soft tissues

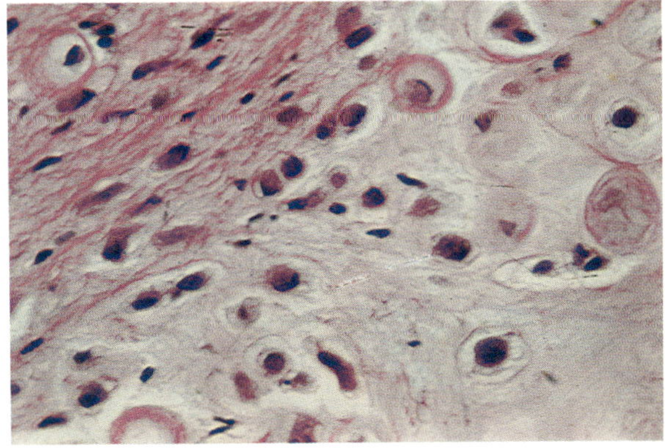

5. Fibrosarcoma of bone

A sarcoma of fibroblasts arising from the medullary cavity and yet producing a large mass in the thigh (**238**).

A thigh cut transversely shows a fibrosarcoma arising from previously normal bone at the lower end of the femur. The cortex is destroyed and the soft tissues are invaded (**239**). Pain, swelling and pathological fracture are the common presenting symptoms. Most fibrosarcomas arise in normal bone, others are associated with Paget's disease, fibrous dysplasia or previous radiation therapy. They are much less common than osteosarcomas.

A well-differentiated cellular fibrosarcoma composed of spindle-shaped malignant fibroblasts (**240** *H&E* × *180*). Mitoses are numerous. There is little collagen production.

Metastases most commonly spread via the blood stream to the lungs. The overall 5 year survival rate is about 30 per cent.

238 Fibrosarcoma of femur

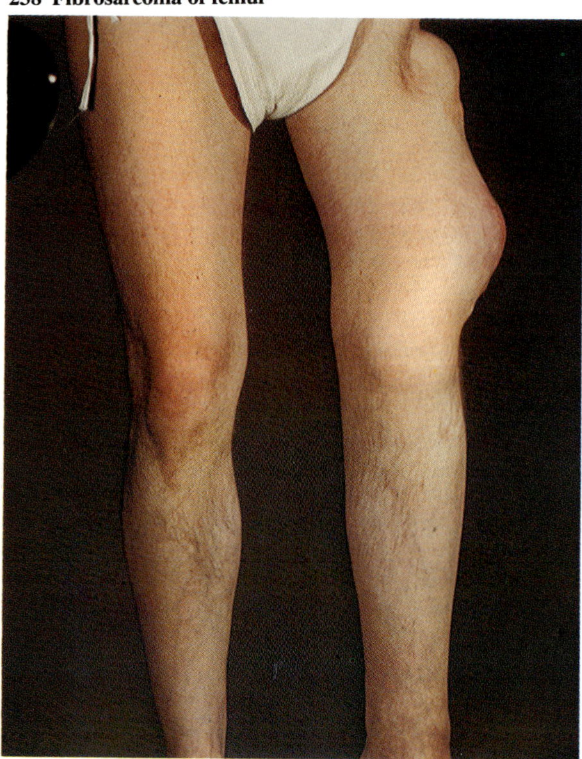

239 Fibrosarcoma of femur

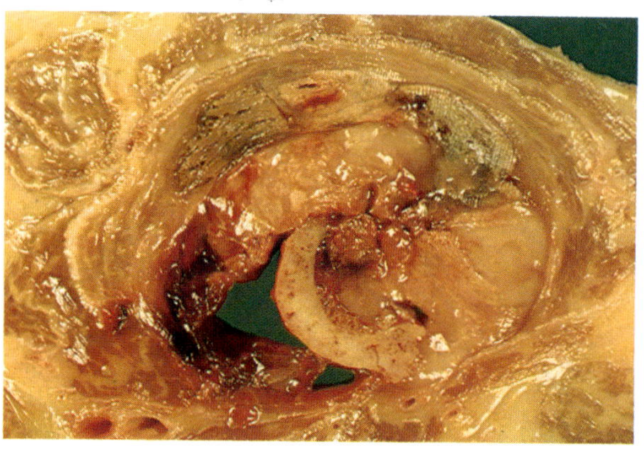

240 Fibrosarcoma

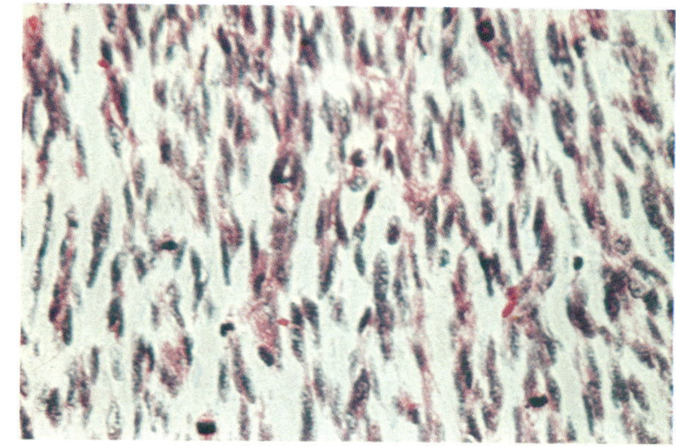

6. Giant cell tumour of bone

Giant cell tumour of bone is a destructive benign or malignant neoplasm arising from non-bone forming stromal tissue. See **241** for distribution.

Giant cell tumour in the skeleton is a brownish, vascular tumour, seen in **242** in the lower end of the radius. Areas may be liquified or rendered fibrotic. Most are less than 10 cm in diameter. About 15 per cent of giant cell tumours are malignant and more than half recur after treatment. Clinically the most common complaints are pain, swelling, tenderness and limitation of movement.

On X-ray a giant cell tumour is seen as an expanded translucent lesion bounded by a thin rim of cortex (**243**). Large tumours often perforate the thinned cortex and periosteum and invade adjacent structures. There is no evidence of new bone formation. No characteristic feature is present and it is essential to confirm the diagnosis by biopsy. Giant cell tumour of bone occurs in skeletally mature individuals, the highest incidence being in the third decade.

241 **Giant cell tumour of bone – distribution (shown unilaterally)**

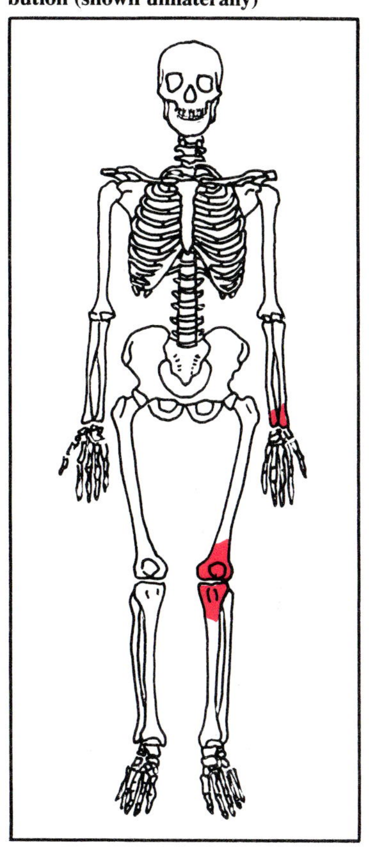

242 **Giant cell tumour of radius**

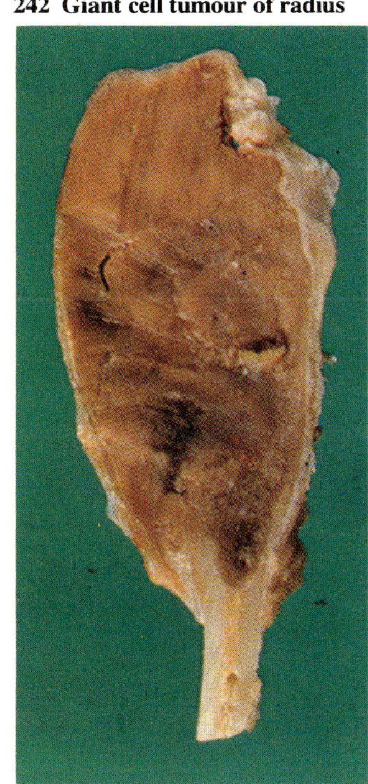

243 **Giant cell tumour of tibia**

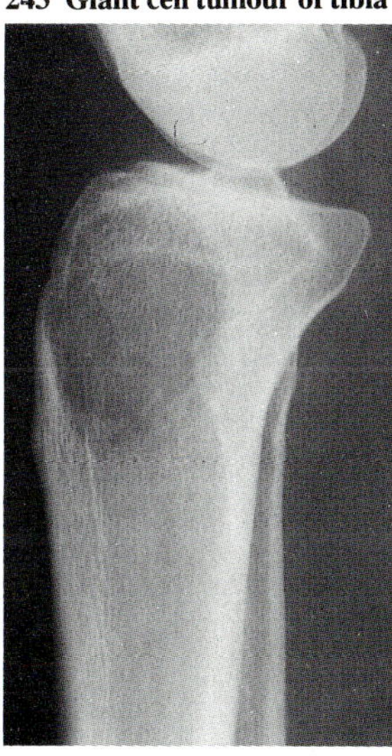

Microscopy shows two elements, multinucleate giant cells and plump ovoid mononuclear cells. Giant cells may be abundant, as in **244** (*demineralised section, H&E × 80*), or scanty. The mononuclear cells are the more important as they determine the behaviour of the neoplasm, which ranges from benign to highly malignant (**245** *demineralised section, H&E × 250*). Histological grading has little prognostic value.

Electronmicrograph of giant cell tumour (**246**). The nuclei of the giant cell (below) and of the ovoid mononuclear cell (above) are similar and it is thought that giant cells probably originate from the fusion of mononuclear cells.

244 **Giant cell tumour**

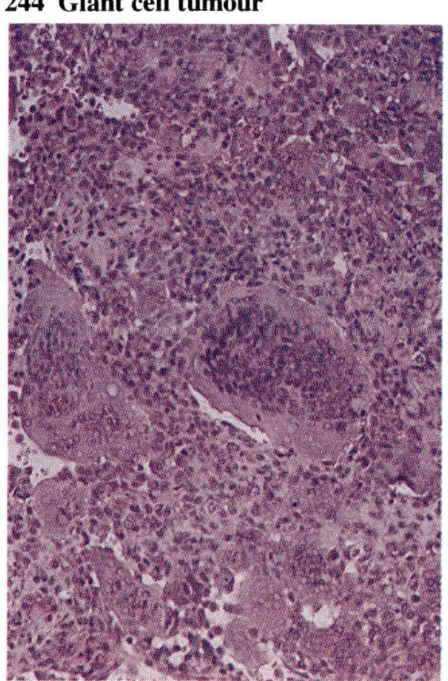

245 **Giant cell tumour**

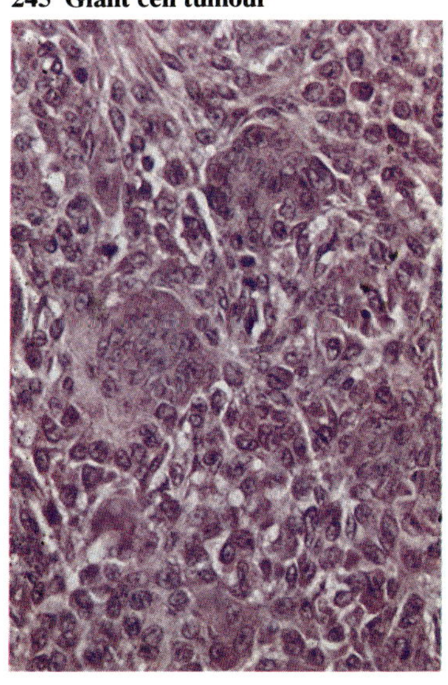

246 **Giant cell tumour**

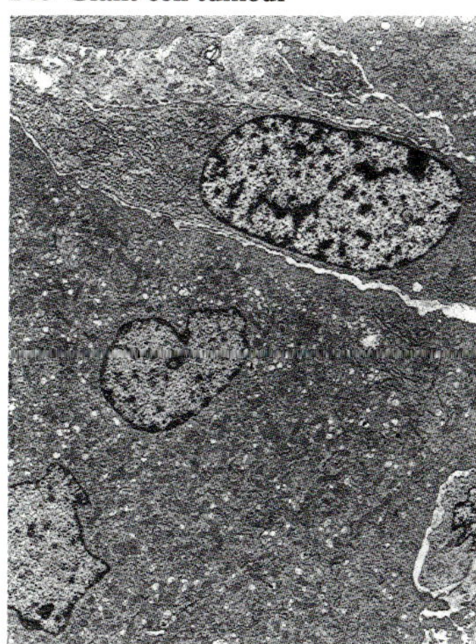

7. Ewing's tumour of bone

Ewing's tumour is an undifferentiated primary tumour of bone. See **247** for distribution.

Early X-ray changes may show only a minor degree of rarefaction and suggest osteomyelitis, but later the presence of a large area of bone destruction combined with a soft tissue mass leaves no doubt as to the existence of a malignant neoplasm. A pathological fracture may be present (**248**).

Microscopically, the neoplasm appears as sheets of fairly uniform, closely applied cells with lightly staining nuclei and indistinct cytoplasmic borders (**249** *H&E × 300*). The presence of PAS positive material in Ewing's tumour cells is helpful in identifying this neoplasm which is often misdiagnosed.

Most patients have micrometastases when first seen and therefore treatment of the primary site alone is unlikely to result in cure.

247 Ewing's tumour – distribution

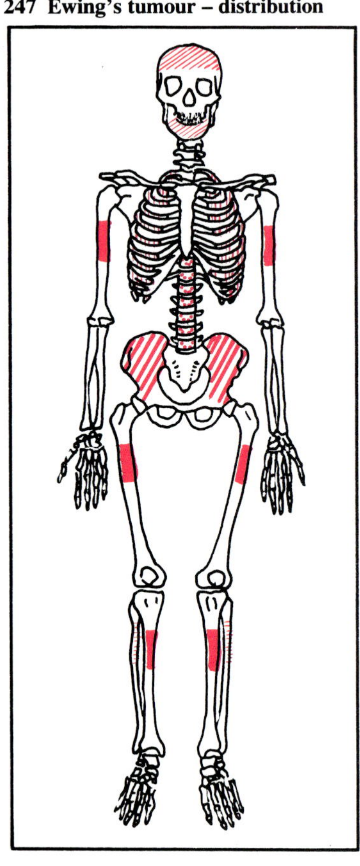

248 Ewing's tumour – pathological fracture

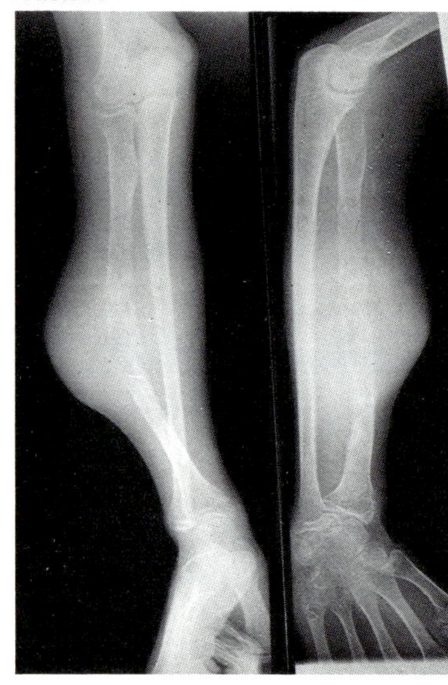

249 Ewing's tumour

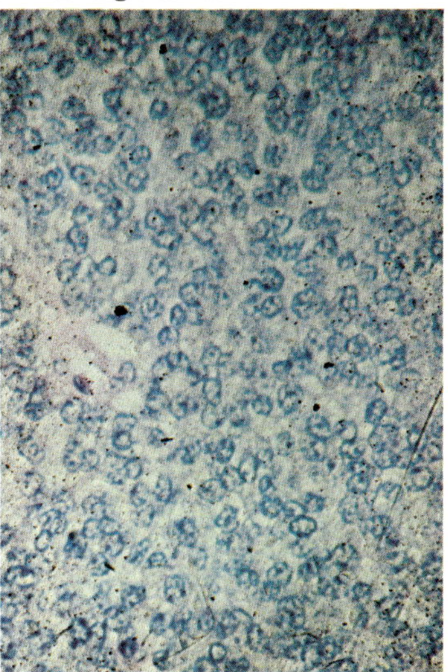

8. 'Adamantinoma' of long bones

Adamantinoma is a rare neoplasm of long bones that occurs most frequently in the tibia. It has an epithelial appearance for which there is no adequate explanation. The common basal epithelial pattern is shown in **250** (*demineralised section, H&E × 250*). Adamantinoma is most common in young adults. It grows slowly and causes pain and local swelling. Recurrence and pulmonary metastasis may follow local excision.

The characteristic radiological appearance is of a well-defined area of translucency with a periosteal reaction, in this case in the radius (**251**). The lesion may be eccentrically placed and involve only part of the cortex.

250 Adamantinoma

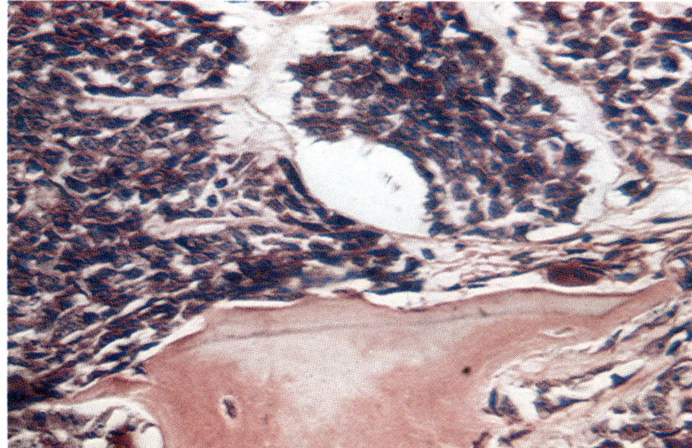

251 Adamantinoma of radius

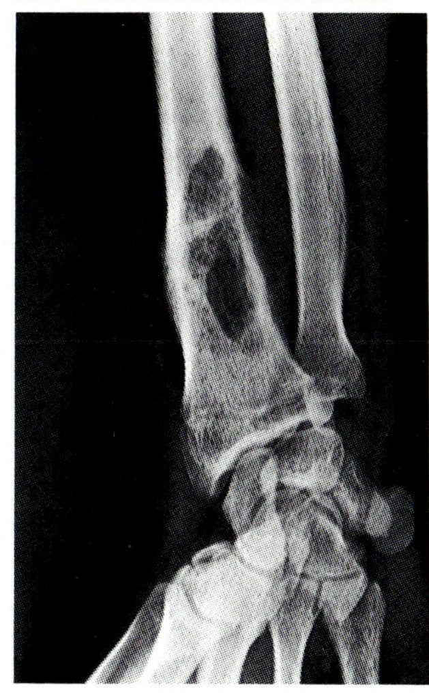

9. Metastases

Bone metastases are much more common than primary malignant bone neoplasms. Almost any primary malignant neoplasm may metastasize to bone, but carcinomas of breast, prostate, lung, thyroid and kidney are the most common. The patient may present with pain, particularly in the spine, a pathological fracture, or symptoms of nerve root or cord compression. Some of the mechanisms are shown in **252**.

252 Mechanisms of metastatic bone disease

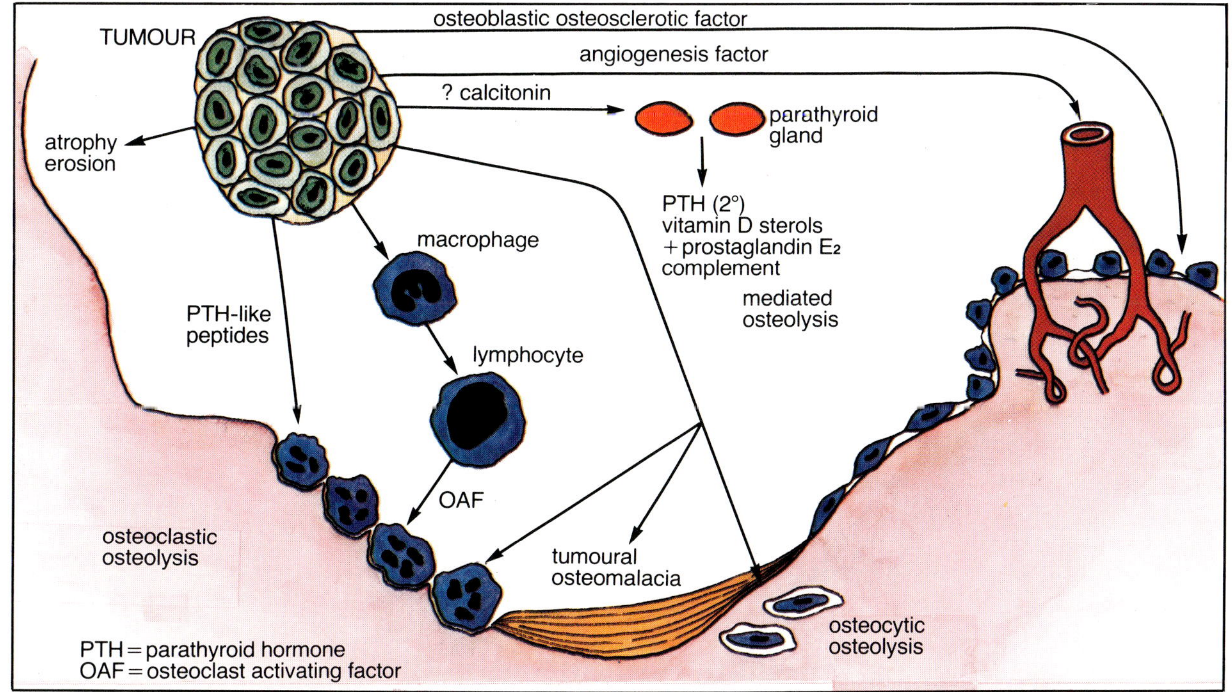

A breast cancer metastasis in the lower end of the femur is seen in sharp contrast to the vascular marrow (**253**). Metastases of this type involve haemopoietic marrow, and if extensive may give rise to leucoerythroblastic anaemia.

Bone metastases are usually multiple. Only rarely can the type of the primary neoplasm, in **254** a malignant melanoma, be diagnosed from the gross appearance. Metastases such as these arise by blood-stream spread of malignant cells that have passed through the lungs. However, some vertebral metastases probably result from retrograde venous spread along the intervertebral plexus of veins.

Most metastases destroy bone and are described as lytic (**255** *demineralised section, H&E × 300*). This type of lesion is readily differentiated from a primary bone neoplasm except when the carcinoma cells assume a spindle shape.

Some metastases, especially from carcinoma of the prostate, promote new bone formation and are described as sclerotic. These may co-exist with lytic lesions. In a scan of both feet (**256**) sclerotic secondaries from carcinoma of the prostate show up as hot red spots.

Metastases from carcinoma of the ovary show erosion of a bony trabecula (**257** *demineralised section, H&E × 250*).

Bone scanning using radioactive isotopes may be used to identify bone metastases. A Tn^{99} EHDP scan of the skeleton shows metastases in the ribs, spine and skull (**258**).

Widespread secondary deposits from carcinoma of the breast are compatible with only moderate symptoms. The only symptoms this patient had were a limp and discomfort, extensive changes subsequently being visible in pelvis radiography (**259**). Supportive surgery can often help and healing of such fractures is quite common.

253 Metastasis from breast carcinoma

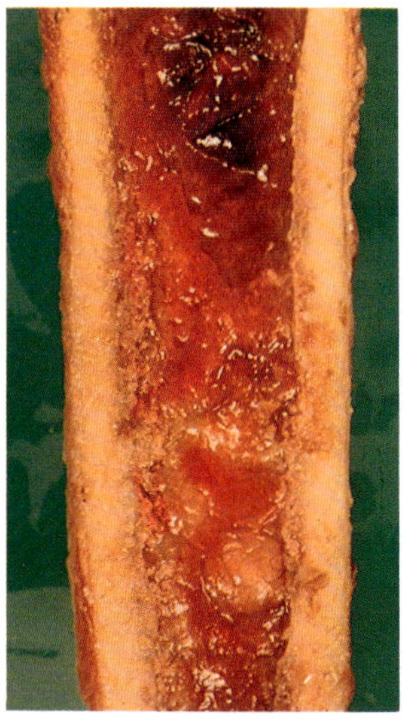

254 Metastases from melanocarcinoma

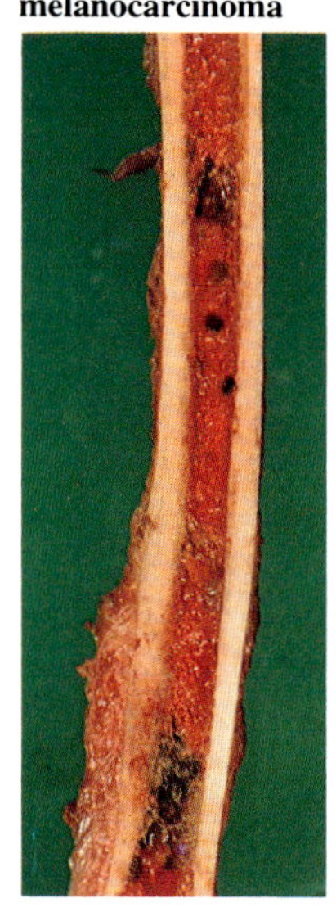

255 Osteolytic metastasis

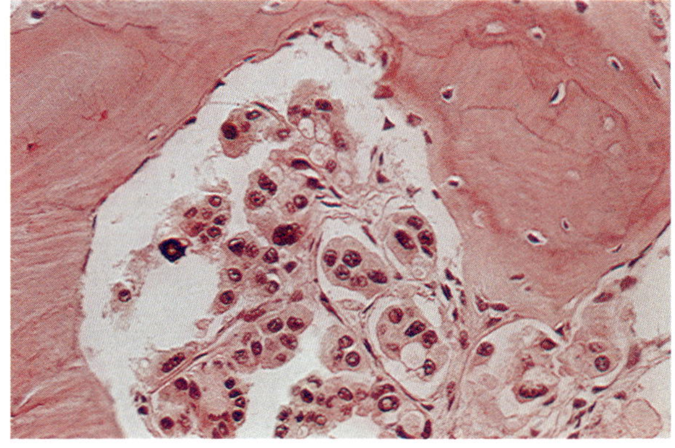

256 Metastases from prostatic carcinoma

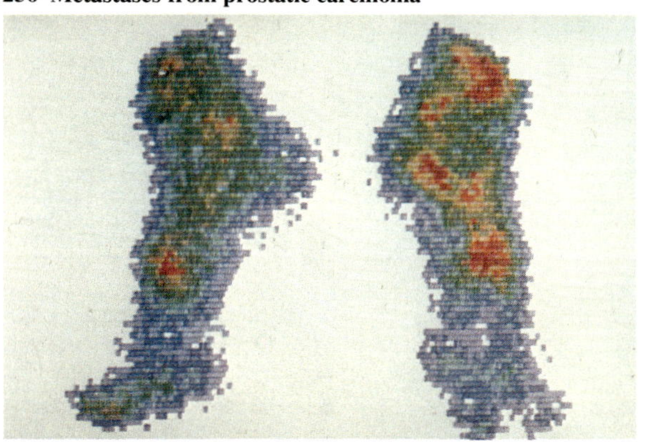

257 Metastases from ovarian carcinoma

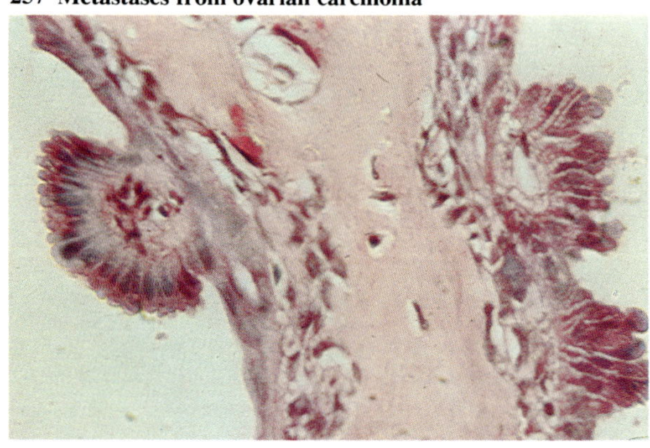

258 Skeletal metastases

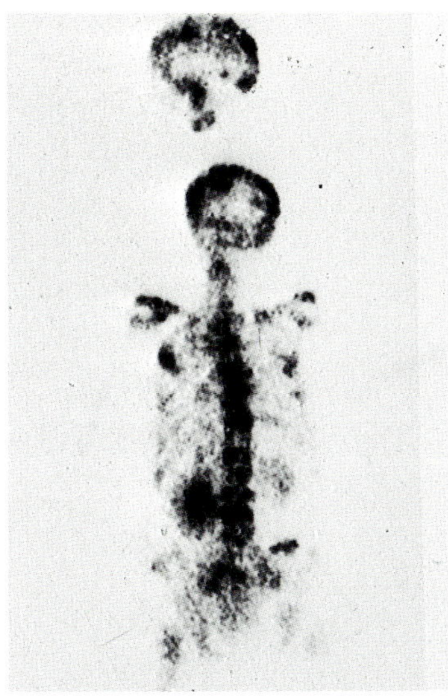

259 Metastases from breast carcinoma

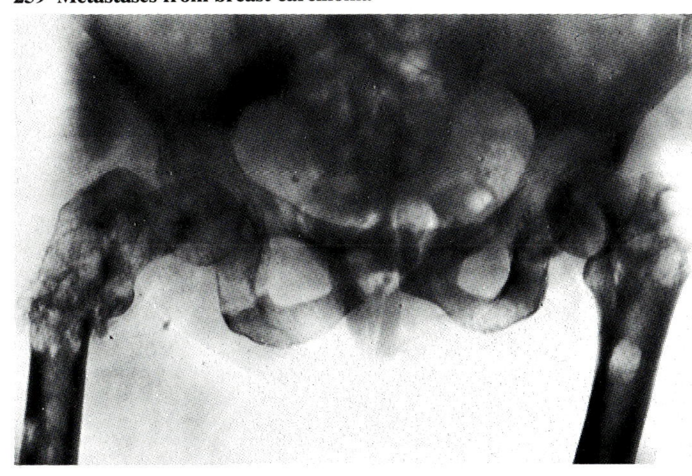

c. Malignant tumours of marrow elements

1. Multiple myeloma

An increase of immunoglobulins arising from a single clone of antibody cells, sometimes referred to as M-components, is characteristic of a number of diseases classified as monoclonal gammopathies, including multiple myeloma and plasmacytoma. Multiple myeloma is a malignant disease of one particular cell of the immune system, the plasma cell.

The osteolytic lesions of multiple myeloma have a discrete 'punched-out' appearance as seen in **260** at the base of the skull. Any part of the skeleton may be involved, but the skull, ribs, sternum, vertebrae, pelvis and proximal limb bones are the most common sites.

The classic translucent 'punched-out' lesions are a characteristic radiological finding (**261**). About 5 per cent of patients present with osteoporosis due to a diffuse infiltration of the marrow by myeloma cells (**262**).

260 Myelomatosis of skull

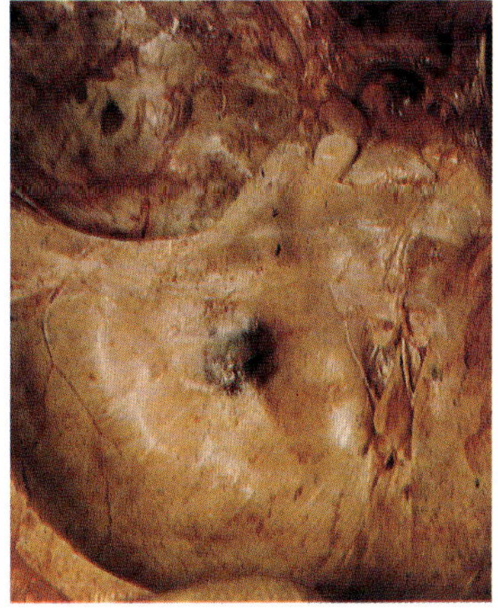

261 Myelomatosis of skull

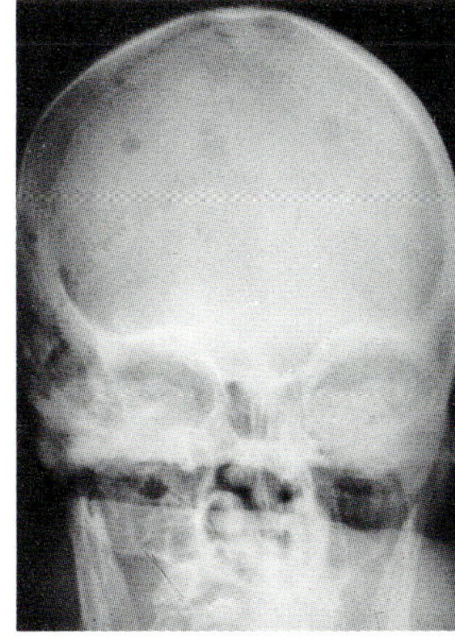

262 Diffuse myelomatosis of skull

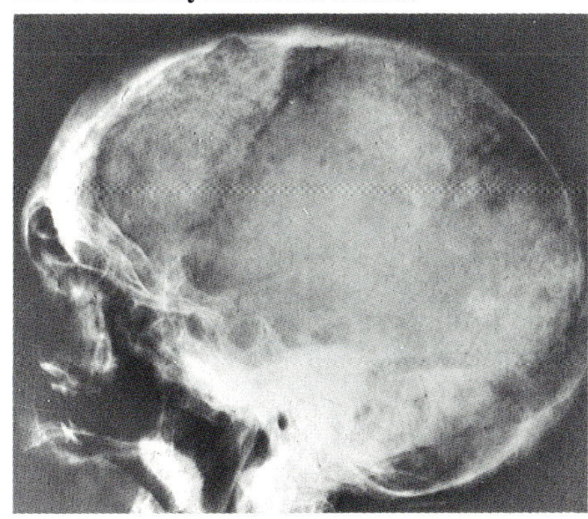

Microscopically, the principal component of the lesion is usually the mature plasma cell (**263** and **264** *H&E × 250 and × 450*). This can be identified by its abundant basophilic cytoplasm, the eccentric nucleus and the deeply stained clumps of chromatin radially arranged around the nuclear membrane. However, these distinctive characteristics are not always present and the cells may be atypical and pleomorphic.

The disease progresses relentlessly to destroy the skeleton and replace both the skeleton and the marrow with soft reddish haemorrhagic masses of myeloma tissue as shown in the humerus in **265**.

A variety of renal lesions may be present but the most common is myeloma kidney which is enlarged, pale and waxy (**266**). Microscopically, many tubules are blocked by proteinaceous casts generally regarded as precipitated Bence-Jones protein. The casts are associated with multi-nucleated giant cells which may partially enclose them (**267** *H&E × 120*).

263 Myeloma cells

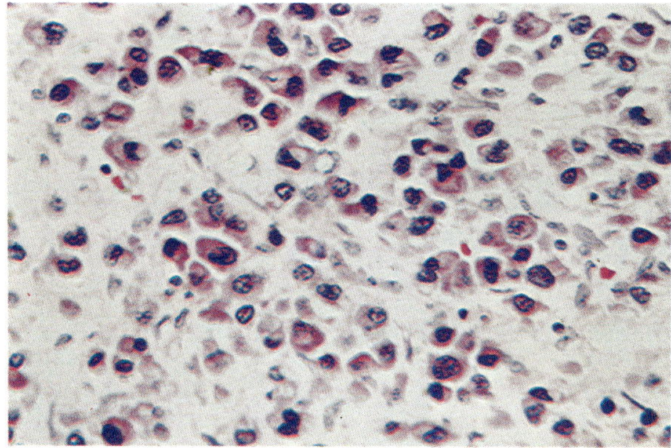

264 Myeloma cells

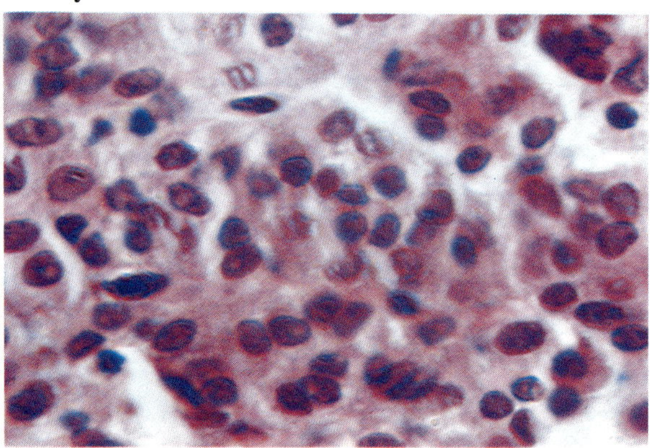

265 Myeloma tissue in humerus

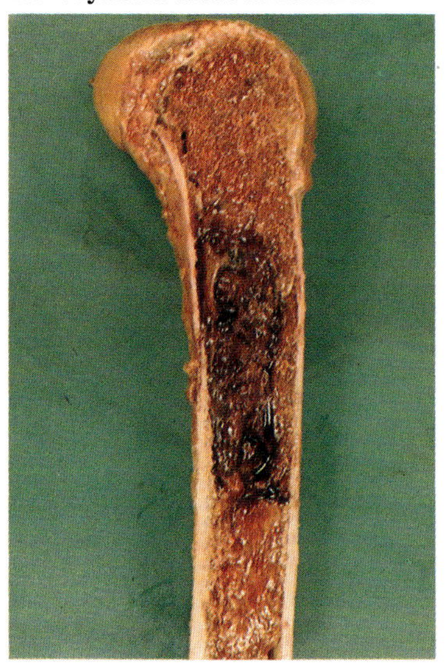

266 Myeloma kidney

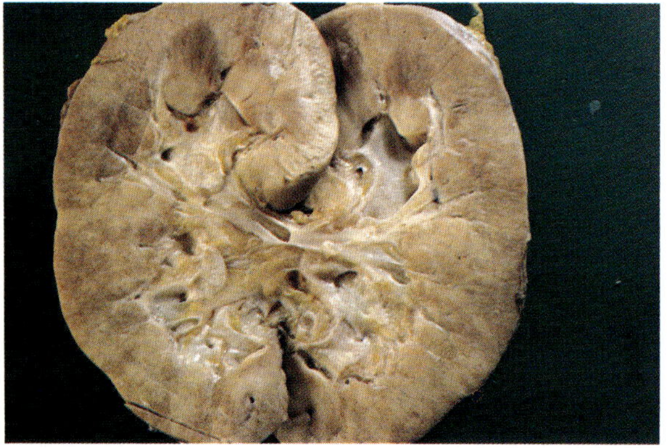

267 Myeloma kidney – casts

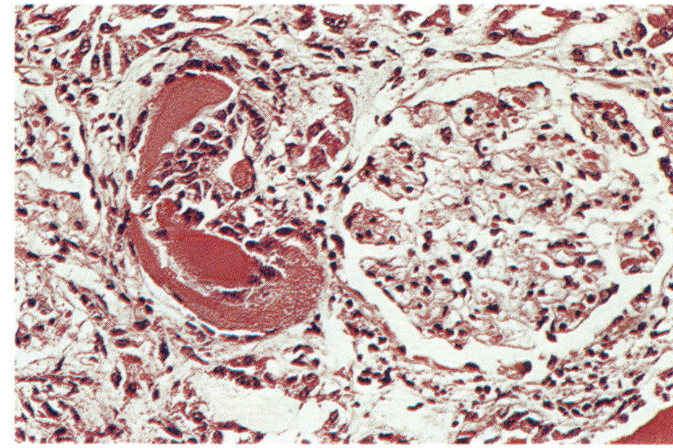

Other lesions which may be present include plasma cell infiltrates in the interstitial tissue, metastatic calcification and amyloid.

An important feature of the disease is the production by the clone of malignant plasma cells of quantities of unique immunoglobulin. These monoclonal proteins (M-components) are present in the plasma as one of the main types of immunoglobulin usually, as in **268**, IgG and its subtypes, sometimes IgA and very occasionally IgM, IgD or IgE.

Electrophoretic strip of concentrated urine showing Bence-Jones protein which appears in the urine of some patients (**269**). This protein is an immunoglobulin polypeptide chain of low molecular weight and therefore able to pass the glomerular filter. It is produced by the clone of malignant cells. Bence-Jones protein appears when the urine is heated to 55° to 60° centigrade if the pH is adjusted to 5. It redissolves if heating is continued and reappears on cooling. Electrophoresis of concentrated urine is a more reliable test for the presence of this protein.

The prognosis in multiple myeloma is poor in spite of chemotherapy; few cases are alive 5 years after diagnosis. Because of the involvement of the lymphoreticular system and defective immune responses, infection, especially bronchopneumonia, is common and not infrequently the terminal event. About 10 per cent of patients with myelomatosis develop amyloidosis.

In a few patients the myeloma lesion is solitary and referred to as a plasmacytoma. The neoplasm generally occurs in bone, as in **270** (in this case a rib), but occasionally the upper respiratory tract or other soft tissues are affected. Myeloma proteins are low or absent and the serum concentrations of non-myeloma immunoglobulins are usually normal. The prognosis is good with a median survival of 8 years.

Under therapy with cytotoxic drugs and fluoride, new bone formation can be demonstrated near the lesions as occurs in this metacarpal (**271**).

268 Myeloma band (top) and normal serum

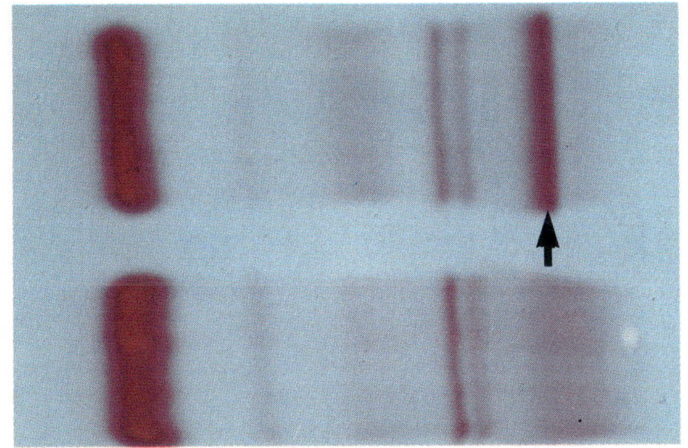

270 Plasmacytoma in rib

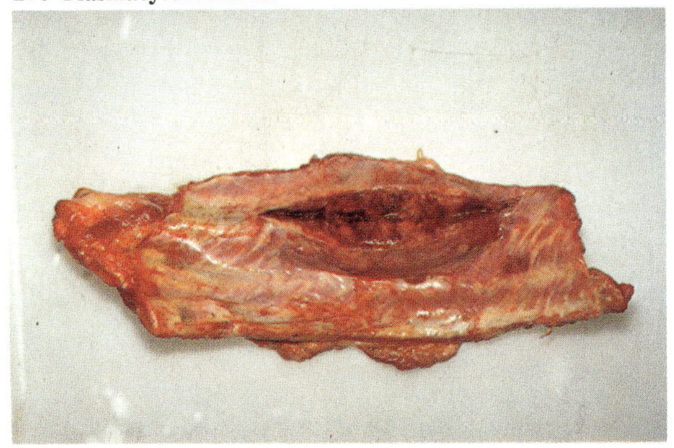

269 Bence-Jones protein

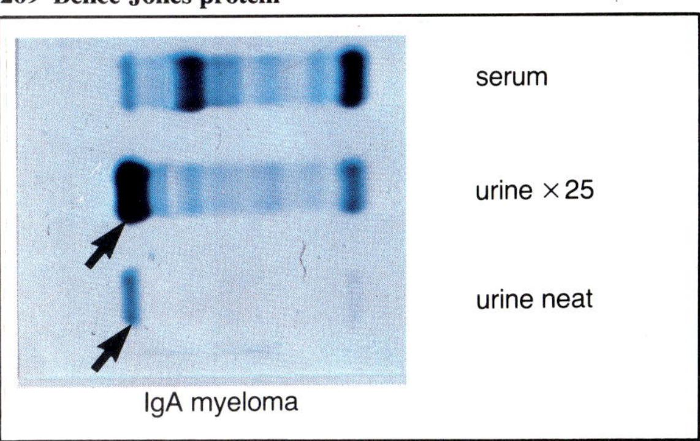

271 Myelomatosis – new bone formation

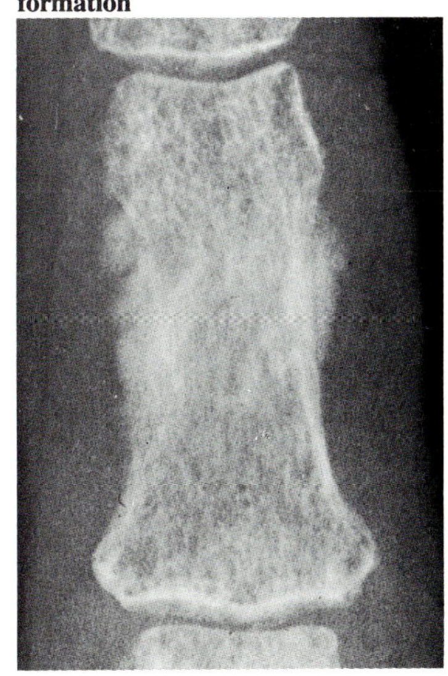

2. Histiocytosis X

Eosinophilic granuloma of bone, Hand-Schüller Christian disease and Letterer-Siwe disease constitute a group of interrelated conditions of which the common factor is a proliferation of cells of the monocyte macrophage series. The term 'Histiocytosis X' relates to the unknown aetiology of the disease process. Eosinophilic granuloma is a localised, benign form of the disease, Hand-Schüller-Christian disease is a more severe and chronic type, and Letterer-Siwe disease is a generalised rapidly fatal form.

i. Eosinophilic granuloma of bone is a rare lesion found predominantly in older children and young adults. It appears as a locally destructive lesion in bone without visceral involvement. Microscopically, the lesion consists of macrophages which may contain lipid, giant cells, eosinophils and polymorphonuclear leucocytes (**272** *H&E* × *200*). The prognosis is excellent, nevertheless a few cases may progress to Hand-Schüller-Christian disease. Unifocal or multifocal osteolytic lesions are seen on X-ray. The flat bones (the skull, mandible, scapula and clavicle) are most commonly involved (**273**).

ii. The classic form of Hand-Schüller-Christian disease consists of foci of bone destruction in the skull (**274**), exophthalmos and diabetes insipidus. Lesions are also found in other bones, the viscera and the skin. Microscopically the lesion is a granuloma similar to eosinophilic granuloma of bone, but the macrophages are rendered foamy by a high cholesterol content (**275** *H&E* × *250*).

iii. In Letterer-Siwe disease, the acute rapidly fatal form of Histiocytosis X, the lesions are predominantly visceral. Skeletal lesions, seen as localised areas of bone destruction, occur mainly in the skull.

272 Eosinophilic granuloma of bone

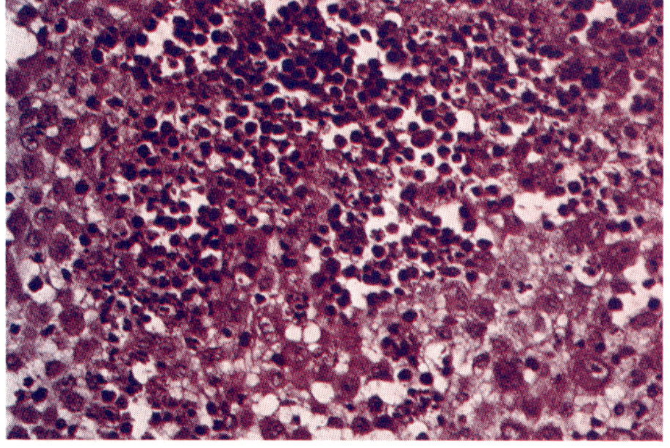

273 Eosinophilic granuloma of bone

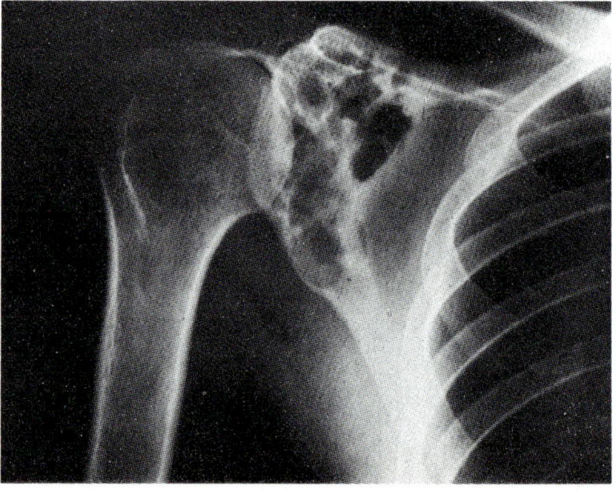

274 Hand-Schüller-Christian disease

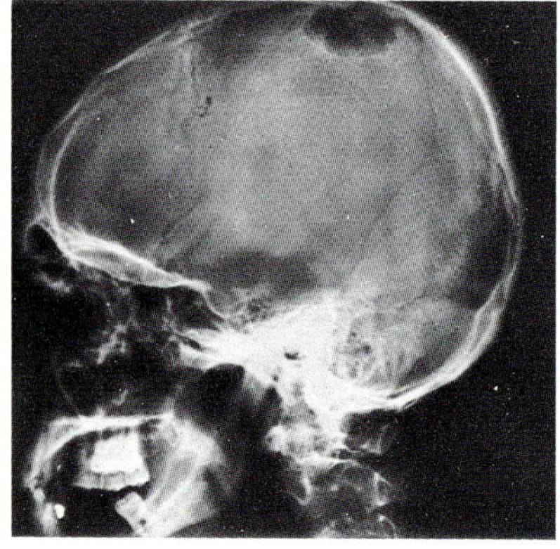

275 Hand-Schüller-Christian disease

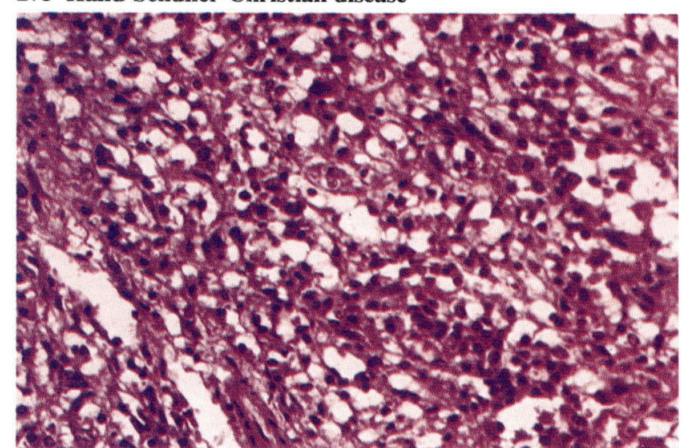

3. Lymphomas

Lymphomas are malignant neoplasms of lymphoreticular tissues. They originate either from lymphoid cells or cells of the monocyte-macrophage series. Since these cells are ubiquitous, lymphomas may occur at any site including the bone marrow. Primary lymphoma of bone is rare and most neoplasms of the group are secondary to lymphoma of the lymph nodes and other soft tissues. They are most common in the elderly. The clinical presentation is with pain, swelling, disability, and sometimes pathological fracture. The commonest bones affected are the femur, ileum and ribs.

There is no characteristic radiological finding. Extensive bone destruction gives the bone a patchy or mottled appearance. New bone formation causes sclerosis and thickening of the cortex which may be mistakenly diagnosed as Paget's disease of bone or chronic osteomyelitis. There is often soft tissue extension, sometimes with calcification.

The lesions are morphologically identical to their lymph node and soft tissue counterparts and may be conveniently grouped as Hodgkin's disease and non-Hodgkin lymphomas.

Non-Hodgkin lymphomas are grouped as follicular or diffuse. The diffuse form includes a large blast cell type usually described as reticulum cell sarcoma (histiocytic lymphoma). See **276** for distribution. This is characterised by pale uniform cells with vesicular nuclei which may be indented and bean shaped. Nucleoli are prominent and the cytoplasm scanty (**277** and **278** *H&E × 300 and × 700*). Reticulin fibres are intimately related to the cells. The prognosis for reticulum cell sarcoma of bone is unexpectedly good: 5 year survival rates of 50 per cent have been reported.

276 Reticulum cell sarcoma – distribution

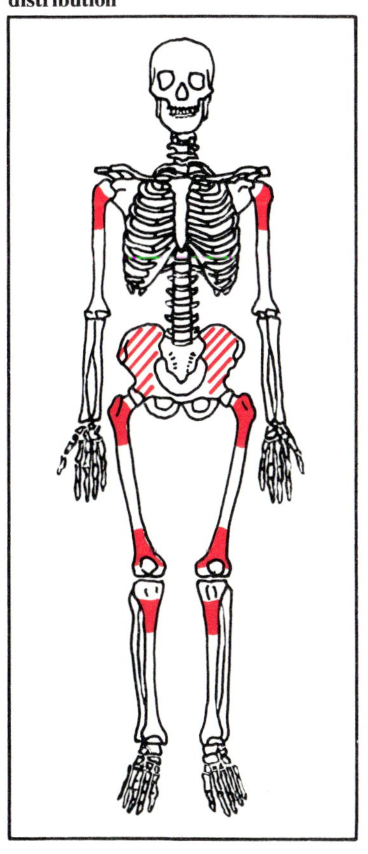

277 Reticulum cell sarcoma of bone

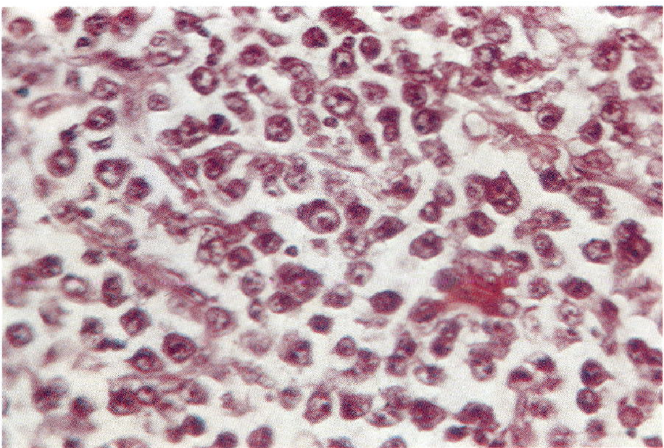

278 Reticulum cell sarcoma of bone

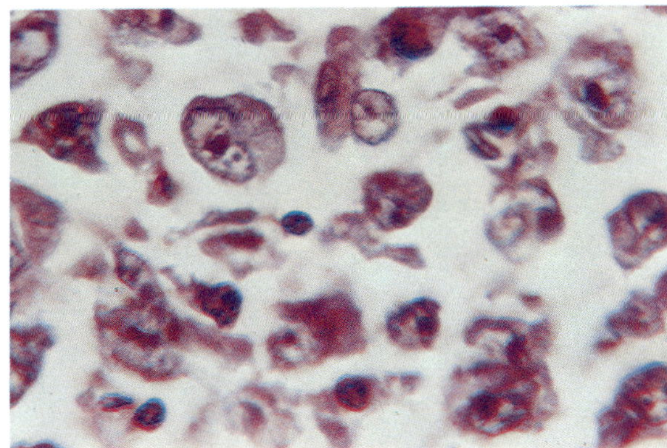

In the classic form of Hodgkin's disease the normal bone structure when seen microscopically is replaced by Sternberg-Reed cells, reticulum cells, lymphocytes, plasma cells and eosinophils together with fibroblasts and abundant reticulin fibres (**279** and **280** *H&E × 250 and × 350*). This picture may be modified to a lymphocytic predominant or lymphocytic depleted type. The prognosis is good for the former but bad for the latter.

279 Hodgkin's disease of bone

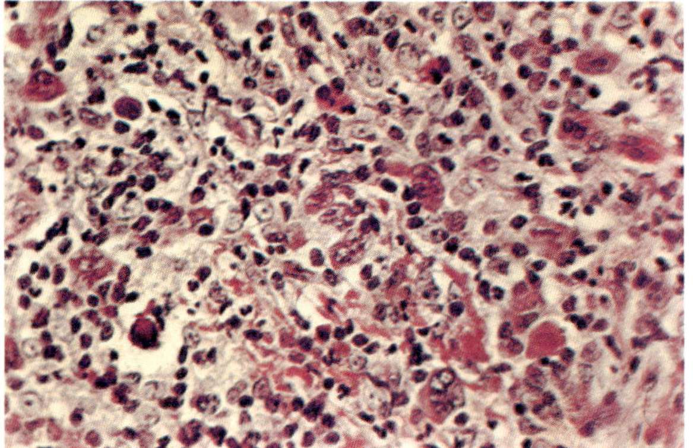

280 Hodgkin's disease of bone

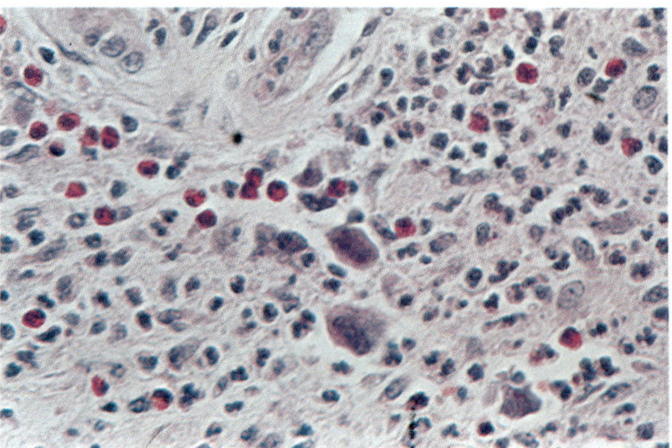

4. Myeloproliferative disorders

The close relationship between bone and its marrow elements is disturbed when the latter proliferate in a variety of conditions. The haemoglobinopathies, sickle cell disease and varieties of thalassaemia lead to increased erythropoiesis in most bones. The skull thickens and cortical bone assumes a fine 'hair on end' appearance. In myelofibrosis the bone marrow is slowly replaced by fibrous tissue and the bones appear denser and haemogeneous. In leukaemia the trabeculae become coarser with patchy lucent areas and periosteal elevation; occasionally gouty changes appear near joints.

5. Bone involvement in systemic disease

a. Congenital disease

1. Achondroplasia

In achondroplasia (**281**), the most common form of dwarfism, endochondral bone formation is retarded but periosteal bone formation proceeds normally. Intelligence and body function are normal so the achondroplastic dwarf is able to lead a normal life. The disease is transmitted as an autosomal dominant.

Achondroplasia is characterised clinically by dwarfism in which short limbs are associated with a large head. The vault of the skull, formed in membrane, is normal, but the bones of the base of the skull are formed in cartilage and as a consequence of restricted growth the forehead bulges and the bridge of the nose is sunken.

Tubular bones are short and appear relatively widened. The epiphyses are inserted in a V-shaped notch in the splayed metaphysis (**282**).

281 Achondroplasia

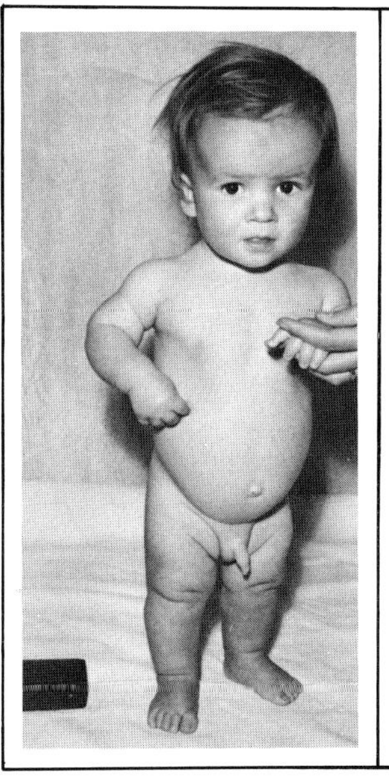

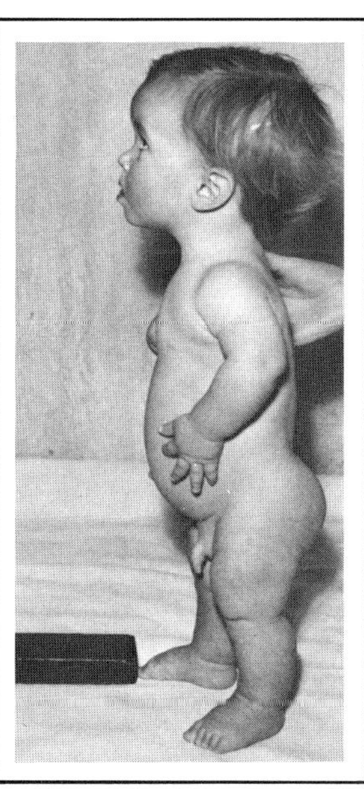

282 Achondroplasia

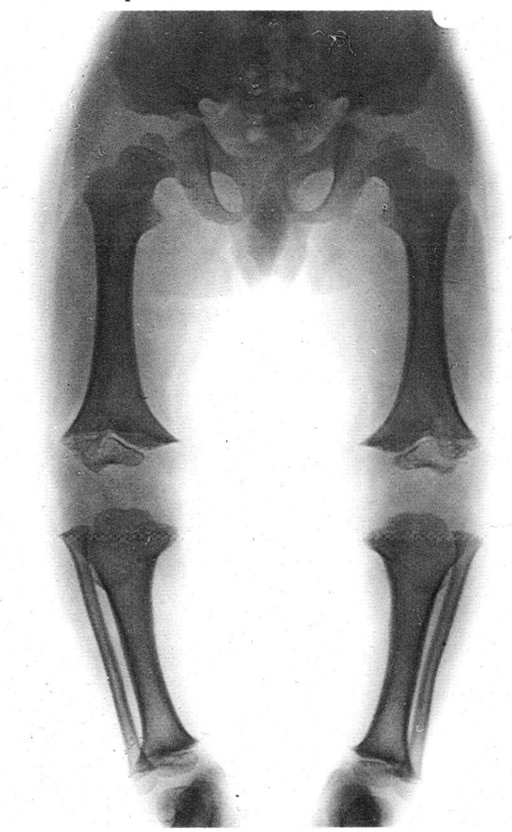

The cartilage cells of the epiphyseal plate form only short rows, are irregularly arranged, and mineralisation is deficient or absent (**283** *demineralised section, H&E × 450*). The decreased rate of endochondral ossification, especially at the epiphyseal growth plates, results in drastic shortening of the long bones of the extremities. The trunk is only a little shortened.

These individuals are prone to two complications: prolapsed invertebral discs and hydrocephalus.

283 Achondroplasia – epiphyseal plate

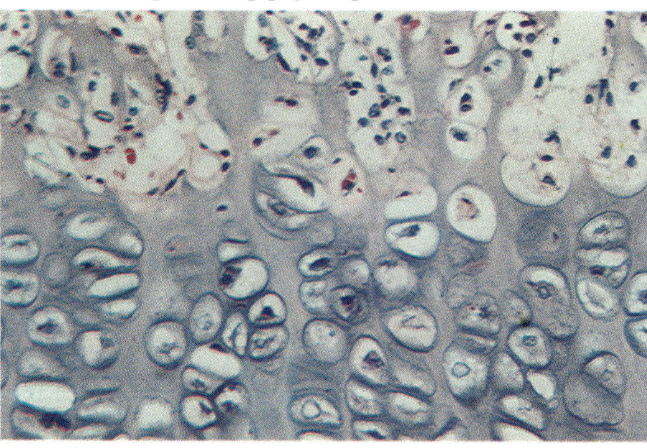

2. Mucopolysaccharidoses and mucolipidoses

These diseases are due to abnormalities of mucopolysaccharide synthesis which involve bone, soft tissue, the lenses of the eye, the nervous system and other organs. Many of them have distinctive clinical and biochemical features but the radiological signs are similar, some developing early in life and others at later ages. See table below.

There are skeletal changes in the skull (large thickened diplöe basal and orbital roofs), the vertebrae (hypoplasia and concavity of all surfaces cause a kyphosis), the ribs and clavicle (thickened and paddle-shaped). The longer bones show shortening of the diaphysis, thickened cortices and the second and fourth metacarpels are shortened and pointed (**284**).

The joints become stiff, mental retardation when it appears is progressive and many children are institutionalised early.

Hepatosplenomegaly is often seen in Hurler's syndrome together with clouding of the cornea.

When laboratory investigations are carried out, the abnormal mucopolysaccharide deposition is seen to be present in many cells, including leucocytes, and in the bone marrow; staining with toluidine blue shows metachromatic granules. Mixed fibroblast cultures from Hurler's and Scheie's syndromes do not each correct the metabolic abnormality in the other, whereas this does occur with other mucopolysaccharidoses.

Mucopolysaccharide (MPS) storage diseases with skeletal involvement

Syndrome	Enzyme deficiency	MPS in urine	Age of onset	Clinical features
Hurler's MPS I.H. 'Gargoylism'	α L iduronidase	Dermatan & Heparan sulphate	first few months	severe skeletal changes, dwarfing, mental retardation, death 10–15 years
Scheie's MPS I.S.	α L iduronidase	Dermatan & Heparan sulphate	later childhood	joint contractions, normal intelligence, normal life expectance
Hunter's MPS II	sulphoiduronate sulphatase	Dermatan & Heparan sulphate	6–12 months	as MPS I.H. but less severe, all patients male
Sanfilippo MPS III	low N Heparan sulphatase or acetyl glucosaminidase	Heparan sulphate	early childhood	mental retardation, joint contractures
Maroteaux-Lamy MPS VI	N-Ac-Gal 4 sulphatase	Dermatan sulphate	early or late childhood	normal intelligence, severe skeletal changes as Hurler's
Morquio's MPS IV	?	Keratan sulphate	2–4 years	normal intelligence, dwarfing, joint laxity

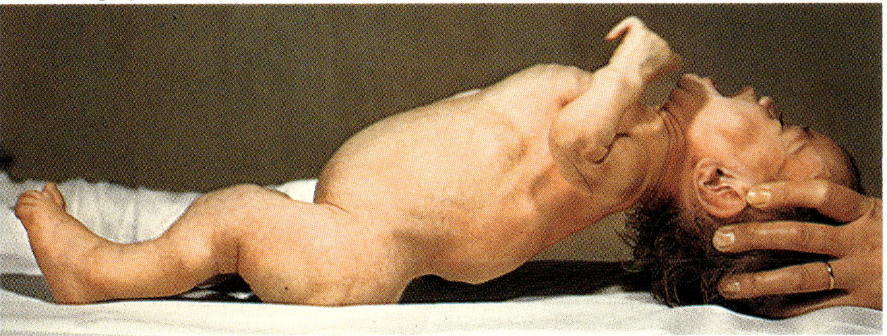

284 Mucopolysaccharidoses

3. Osteogenesis imperfecta (OI)

Osteogenesis imperfecta is an inherited disorder of collagen that results in skeletal and connective tissue defects. The condition may develop during intrauterine life (osteogenesis imperfecta congenita) when it is generally fatal, or later in childhood (osteogenesis imperfecta tarda) when the severity varies.

Trabeculae are small and irregular and they fail to mature to lamellar bone (**285** *demineralised section, H&E × 100*).

285 Osteogenesis imperfecta

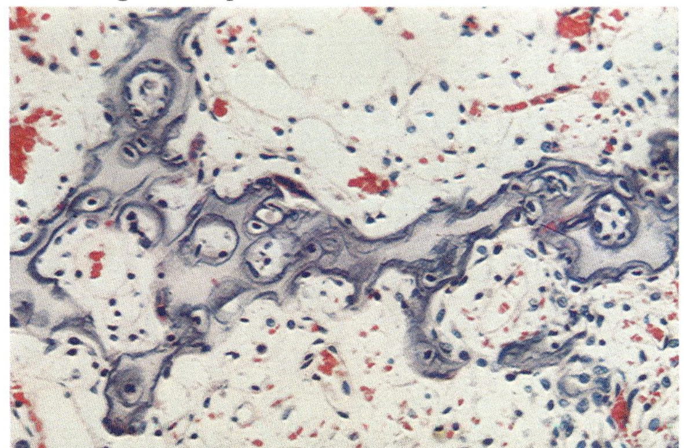

287 Osteogenesis imperfecta – skeletal deformities

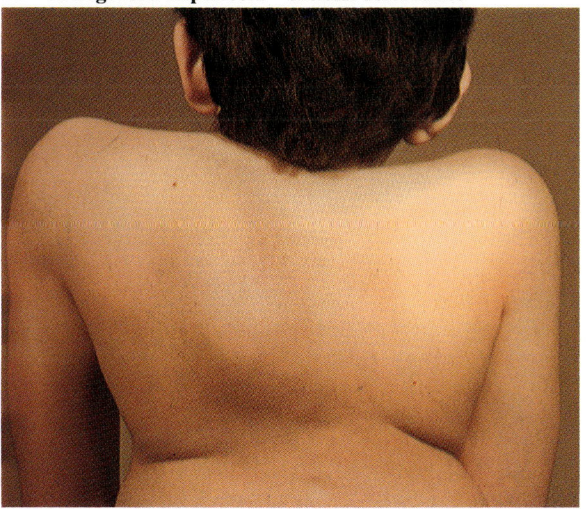

Cortical bone is thin and fragile so that in severe cases the patient is prone to pathological fractures and extreme deformities (**286**). Growth is defective and the sufferer is stunted or dwarfed with shortening of the axial skeleton and limbs. A 16 year old boy with a severe kyphosis (**287**).

The sclerae appear bluish because they are thin and the pigmented choroid shows through (**288**). Thin skin and lax ligaments with joint hypermobility may be present. Dentine is not properly formed and the teeth are discoloured.

The disorder is usually transmitted as an autosomal dominant. The wide range of genetic expression is ascribed to incomplete penetrance of the dominant gene and blue sclerae may be the only manifestation.

286 Osteogenesis imperfecta

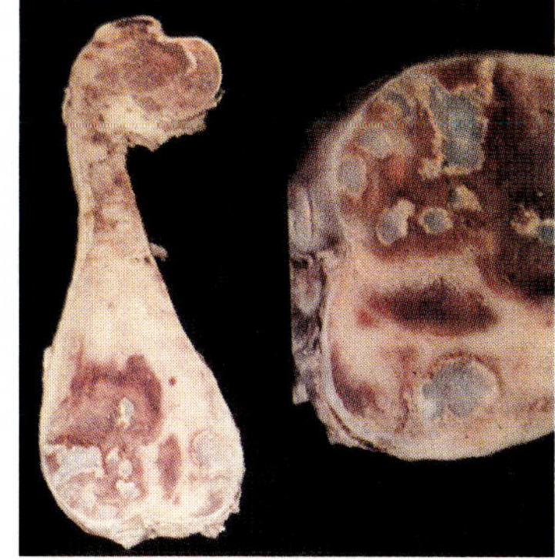

288 Osteogenesis imperfecta – bluish sclerae

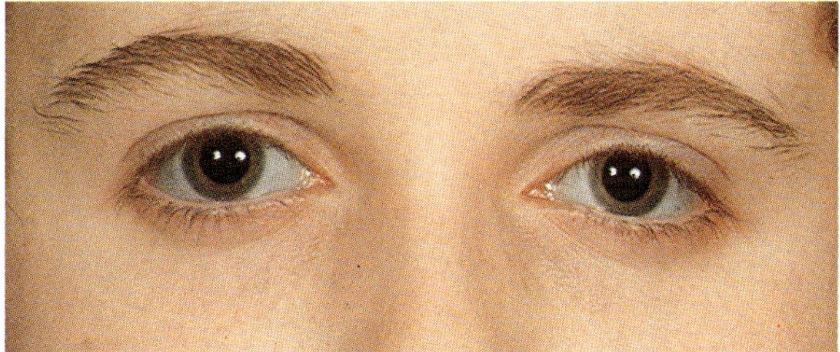

4. Osteopetrosis

Osteopetrosis is characterised by excessive density and thickening of the bones. The severity of the disease varies from mild forms compatible with longevity to the severest forms leading to death in foetal life. The disease is hereditary.

The characteristic picture is of persistent cores of cartilage within thickened trabeculae (**289** *demineralised section, H&E × 200*). Pathological fracture is often a presenting feature. The thickened bone displaces the marrow to give rise to normochromic or even leucoerythroblastic anaemia. Involvement of the skull may result in optic atrophy, facial palsy and other cranial nerve disorders.

5. Gaucher's disease

Gaucher's disease is an inherited disorder of lipid metabolism characterised by the accumulation of glycocerebrosides in the bone marrow, spleen, liver and other organs.

The diagnosis of Gaucher's disease is confirmed by the finding of large foam cells on bone marrow puncture. The ballooned, foamy, Gaucher's cells are reticuloendothelial cells distended by kerasin which gives the cytoplasm a curious ground-glass appearance (**290** *H&E × 450*).

Aggregations of Gaucher's cells in the marrow cause irregular foci of bone destruction. Diffuse displacement of the marrow by Gaucher's cells results in corticol thinning which may lead to pathological fractures. An additional hazard is the pressure of the masses of Gaucher's cells on the blood vessels of the marrow causing infarction of bone.

289 Osteopetrosis – thickened trabeculae

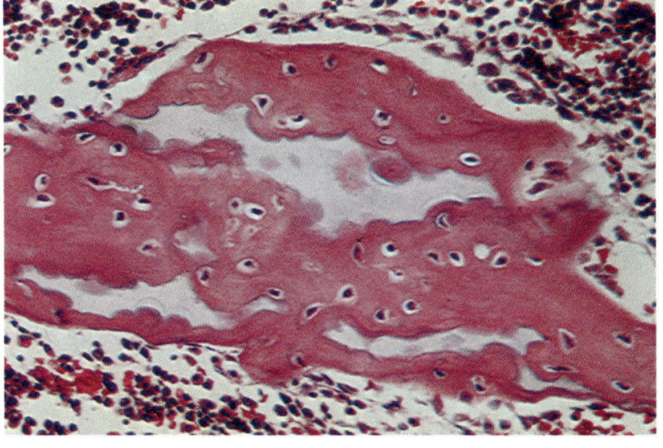

290 Gaucher's disease – foamy cells

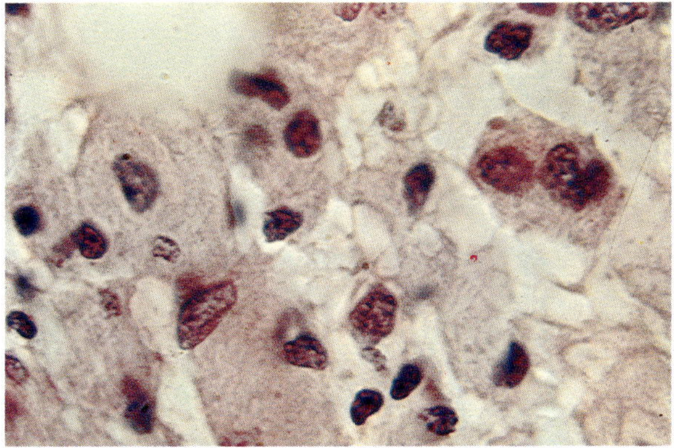

b. Acquired disease

1. Fibrous dysplasia

Fibrous dysplasia is a non-neoplastic condition of unknown aetiology characterised by the replacement of normal bone substance by fibro-osseous connective tissue.

Most fibrous dysplasia lesions are radiolucent with well-defined sclerotic margins as in **291**. Others, depending on the amount of bone formed, are semi-opaque or opaque. Expansion of the affected bone and thinning of the cortices are usual. In patients with multiple lesions it is necessary to exclude hyperparathyroidism.

The bone and bone marrow are replaced by a circumscribed mass of fibrous tissue containing curved spicules of woven bone hedged by osteoblasts (**292** *demineralised section, H&E × 120*). The femur, tibia, ribs, jaw and skull are most frequently affected. The lesions may be single (monostotic) or multiple (polyostotic). See **293** for distribution (monostotic left, polyostotic right). Sarcoma is an extremely rare complication.

When fibrous dysplasia lesions are multiple and associated with café-au-lait pigmented patches in the skin and disturbances of endocrine function, the condition is known as Albright's syndrome. The bone lesions tend to be unilateral and skin pigmentation to be on the same side as the bone lesions. Typical features are shown in **294**, the 'Shepherd's Crook' deformity of the femur in **295** and an excess of osteoid on bone biopsy in **296** (*von Kossa's stain × 60*).

291 Fibrous dysplasia

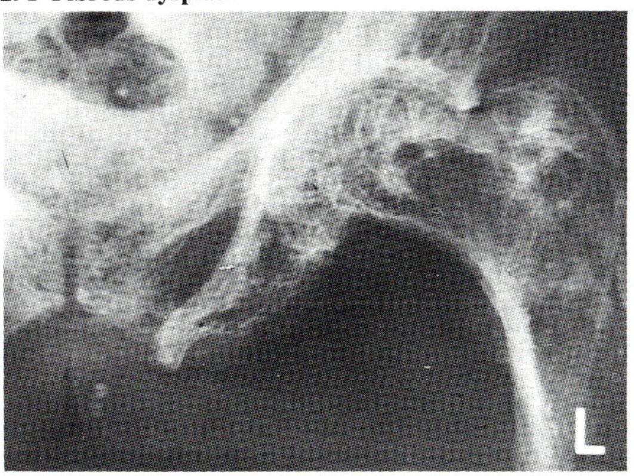

292 Fibrous dysplasia

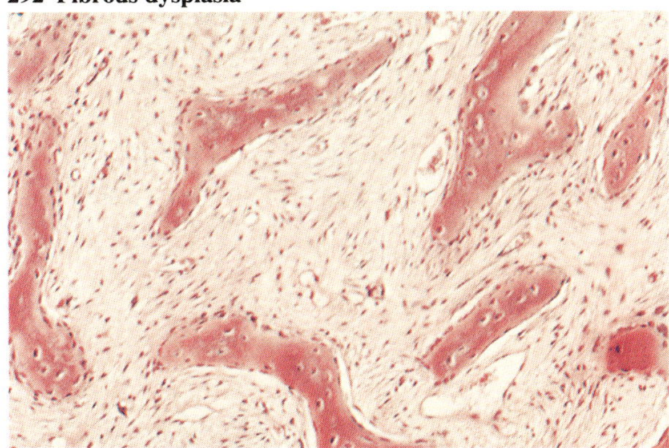

293 Fibrous dysplasia – distribution

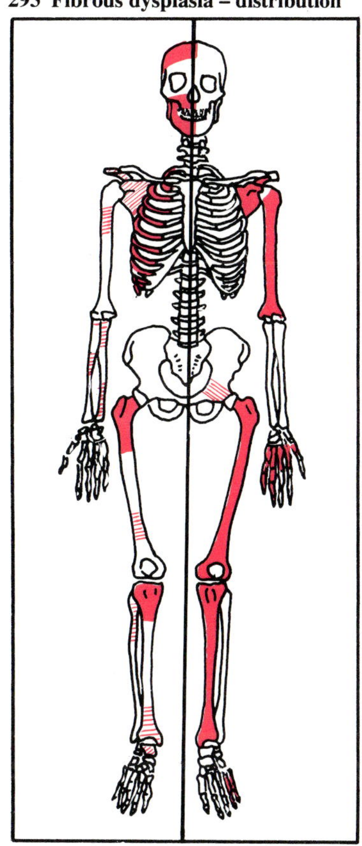

294 Fibrous dysplasia

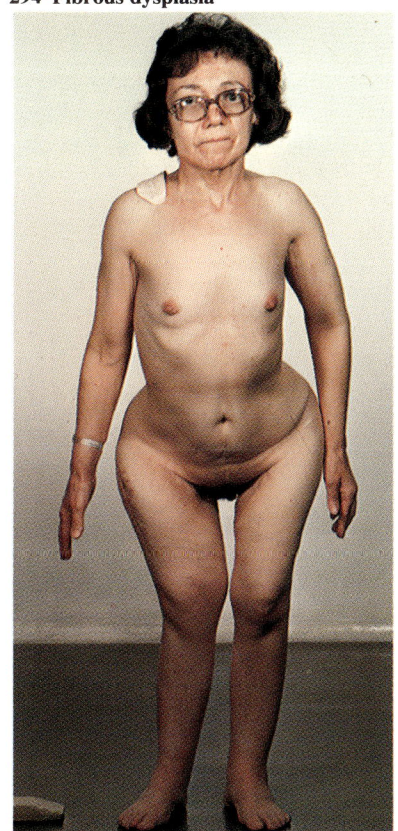

295 Fibrous dysplasia – 'Shepherd's Crook' deformity

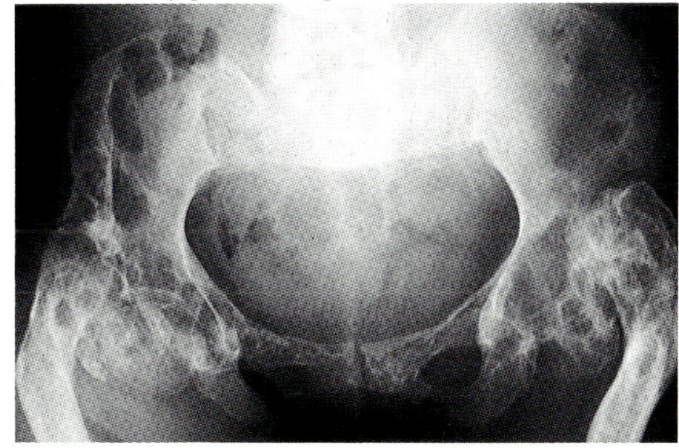

296 Albright's syndrome – excess of osteoid

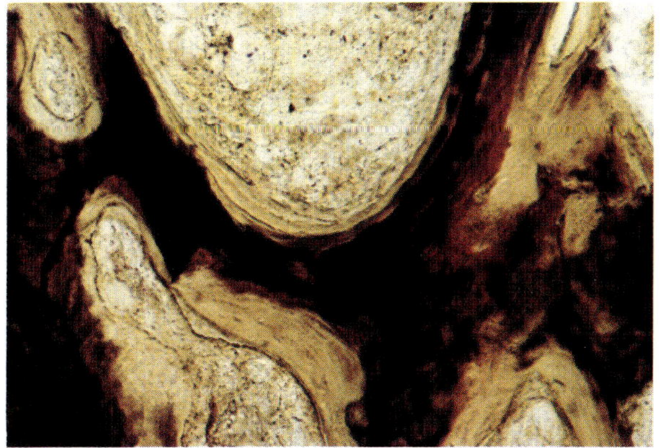

Metaphyseal fibrous defects are benign developmental abnormalities. Large lesions are designated non-ossifying fibroma. They occur in the metaphyseal region of long bones in children.

The radiological appearances are usually distinctive enough for a diagnosis to be made; they include a lobulated elongated translucent area surrounded by a shell of sclerotic bone close to the cortex. If the lesion is large a pathological fracture may result. Many metaphyseal fibrous defects become reossified.

Spindle-shaped fibroblasts intermingled with macrophages and small multinucleated giant cells form the principal component (**297** *H&E* × *150*). Haemosiderin deposits impart a brown colour to the lesion. Occasionally the fibrous defect is mistaken for fibrosarcoma.

297 Metaphyseal fibrous defect

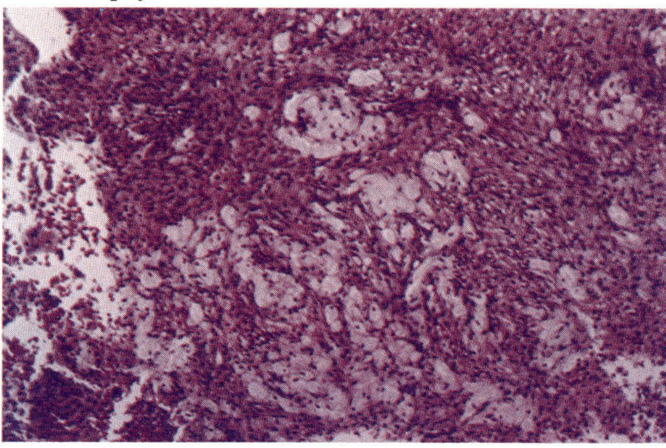

2. The osteochondroses

These conditions affect one or more of the epiphyses leading to a fragmentation and separation of the epiphyseal structures. The underlying microscopical pathology appears to be a degenerative or even necrotic condition stemming from an interference with the epiphyseal blood supply. This may be the result of single or multiple trauma associated occasionally with an obese, Fröhlich type of endocrine upset. The condition can occur with other anomalies of bone growth such as slipping of the epiphysis, renal osteodystrophy and Gaucher's disease. Familial prevalence has been recorded and multiple epiphyses may occasionally be involved.

The following four main sites account for over 70 per cent of cases:

- tibial tuberosity 30% (Köhler)
- calcaneal apophysis 20% (Sever)
- vertebral epiphysis 15% (Schauerman)
- capital femoral epiphysis 7% (Legg-Calvé-Perthes)

Over 40 other sites each with an eponym have been described to make up the total percentage.

Osteochondrosis of the femoral head of a young boy is shown in **298**, **299** and **300**. Fragmentation of the epiphysis and eventual healing is seen at intervals of 2 years.

298 Perthes' disease

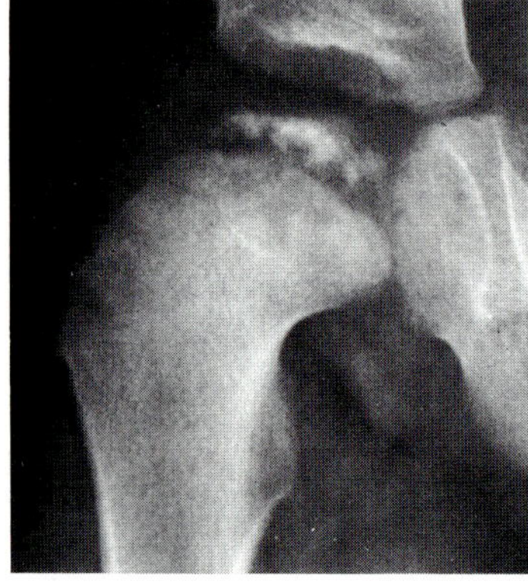

299 Perthes' disease

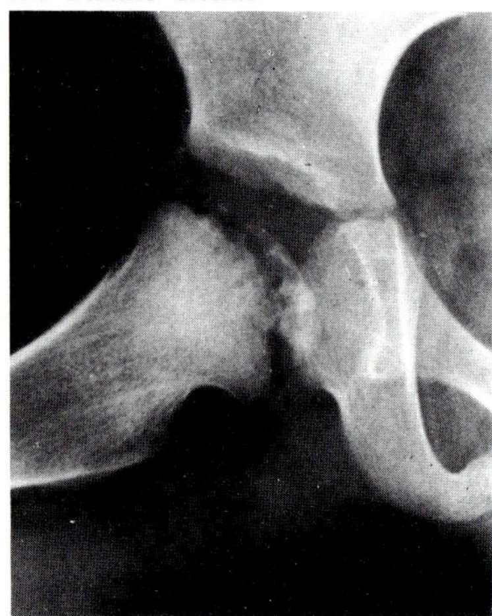

300 Perthes' disease

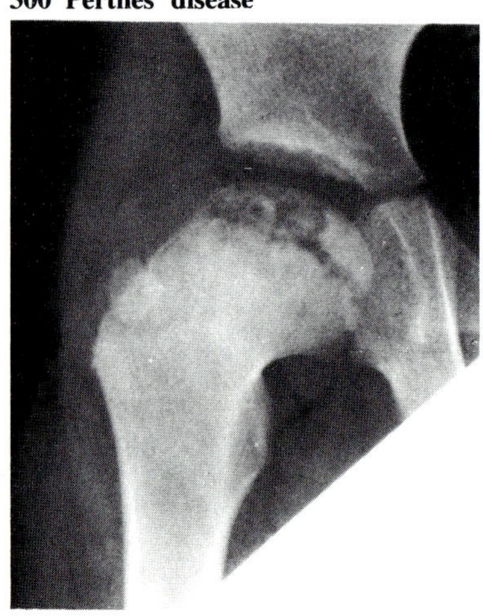

3. Myositis ossificans

The term myositis ossificans refers to the ossification of the connective tissue of muscle. It is a metaplasia that occurs most often, following injury in young active adults, in the anterior and lateral aspects of the thigh.

Ossification first becomes apparent a few weeks after the onset of symptoms (pain, tenderness and sometimes fever). With the passage of time the lesion becomes increasingly apparent radiologically as a spherical mass within muscle (**301** and **302**). The lesion may be mistaken for a parosteal osteosarcoma if the adjacent periosteum is involved or for a soft tissue osteosarcoma.

Microscopy reveals young proliferating fibroblasts and osteoblasts lining trabeculae of osteoid and bone (**303** *demineralised section, H&E × 150*). Cartilage may be present. Characteristically ossification is most pronounced at the periphery of the lesion and is seen as an orderly zonal arrangement not present in osteosarcoma. Adjacent muscle fibres may be atrophied as seen in **304** (*demineralised section, H&E × 150*).

301 Myositis ossificans in hip muscles

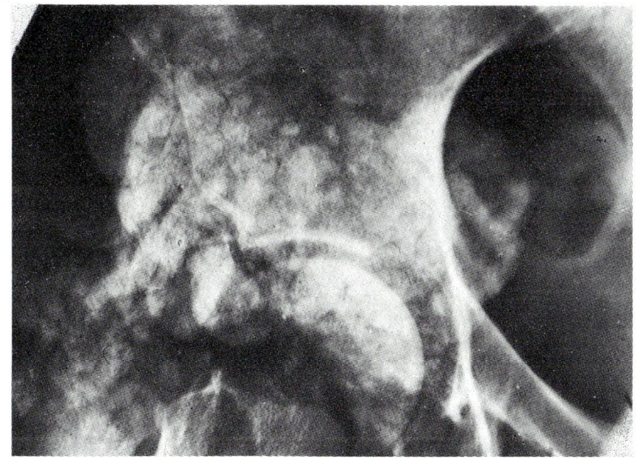

302 Myositis ossificans in muscles around thorax

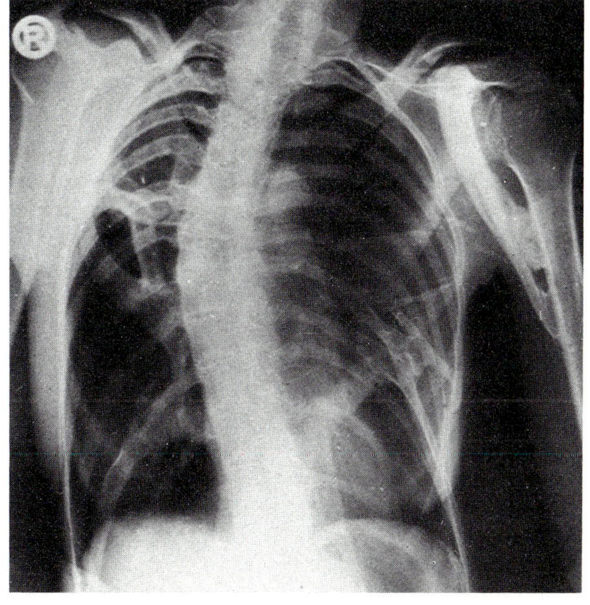

303 Myositis ossificans

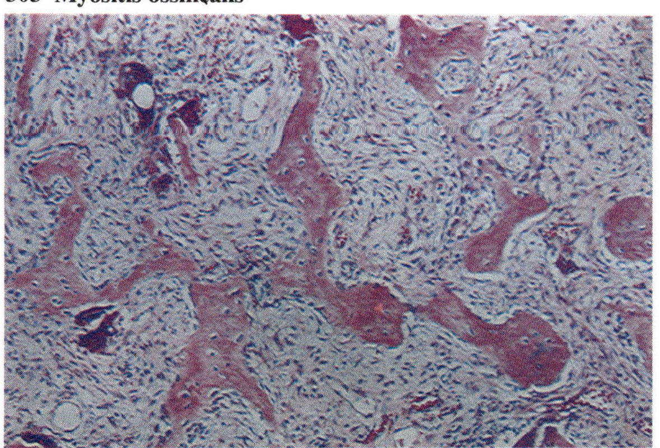

304 Myositis ossificans – atrophic muscle

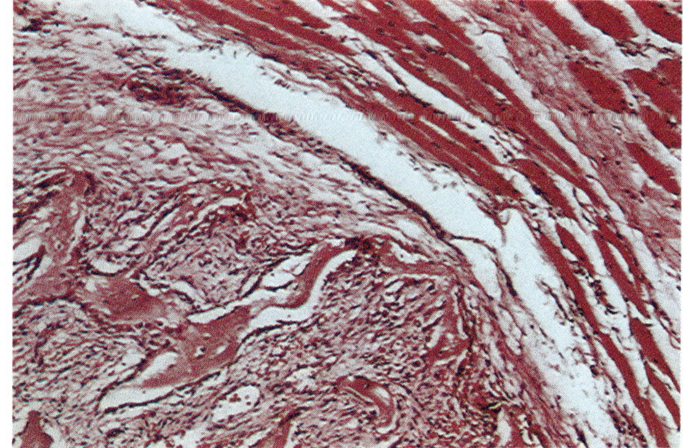

4. Bone disease accompanying joint disease

The differential diagnosis between some types of arthritis is greatly helped by the radiological examination not only of the joints in which the symptoms appear, but also of other joints, for example of the hands. However, many metabolic diseases share similar joint changes and other criteria are required in the diagnosis of these disorders. Only major pathological divisions of the arthridites will be mentioned to illustrate the mechanisms.

Types of arthritis with bony involvement:

i. Traumatic arthritis – bone fractures into the joint fill the joint with haemorrhage, distend the capsule and are followed by effusions. There may also be ligamentous and cartilaginous damage leading to deformity and instability, which in turn lead to degenerative changes later in life.

ii. Septic arthritis – osteomyelitis may extend into the joint, or blood-borne synovial sepsis may more rarely lead to bony involvement (**305**). The organisms commonly involved include staphylococci, pneumococci, streptococci and salmonellae. Sections through the joint show acute inflammatory exudate osteolysis, synovial reaction and occasionally islands of necrotic bone. In chronic infections such as tuberculosis the joint and bone changes are more extensive; they may result in destruction of the joint (**306**).

305 Acute septic arthritis

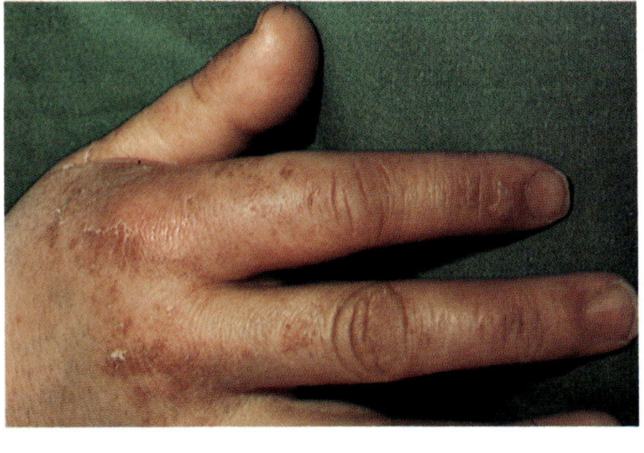

306 Septic arthritis in knee

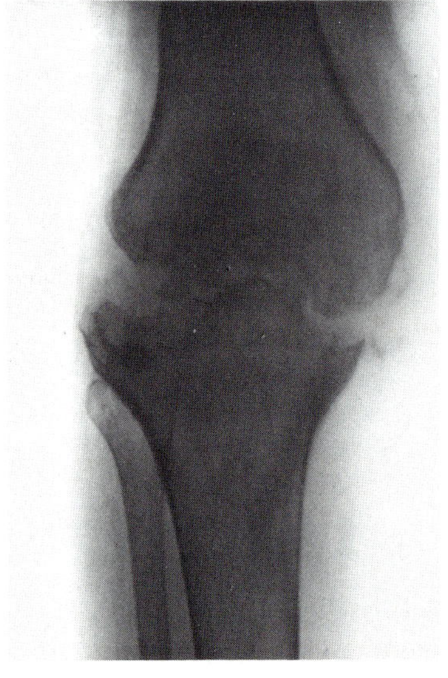

iii. Immunological arthritis

a. Rheumatoid arthritis – this connective tissue disorder involves primarily the synovial, periosteum, tendon sheaths and more rarely the tendons themselves. Synovial joints throughout the body can be affected. Changes in the bone near the affected joints are best seen in the hands (**307**), but they are found in all seriously affected areas. The immunological complexes which lead to synovial proliferation (pannus) migrate through the synovia and can be found in the joint fluid. They set up an inflammatory response which liberates osteolytic collagenases, proteases and permeability factors including prostaglandins into the attachment of synovia to bony periosteum. Complement mediated leucotaxis leads to a further cell migration of leucocytes which together with the synovial cells may be responsible for the prolonged production of collagenases and prostaglandins. The rheumatoid dissolution of bone is seen as:

- invasion of bone by pannus seen on radiology as an erosion (**308**), and microscopically as areas of granulation tissue within bone (**309** *H&E × 65*) and the marrow leading to cyst formation
- an intense cellular infiltrate of chronic inflammatory cells with corresponding proliferation of osteoclasts and osteocytes (**310** *H&E × 25*)
- destruction of bony trabeculae and the collapse of normal cortical and medullary architecture
- rheumatoid nodules may form along the periosteum
- cartilage destruction by pannus occurs and the articular surfaces become irregular showing some of the changes of osteoarthrosis (**311**)
- disuse atrophy of bone (osteoporosis)

307 Rheumatoid arthritis

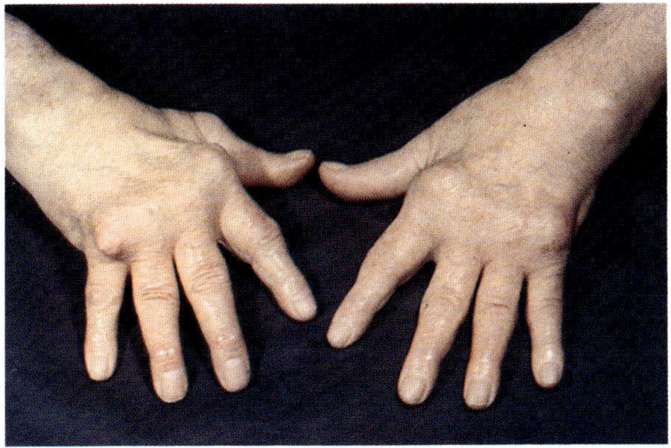

308 Rheumatoid arthritis – invasion of bone by pannus

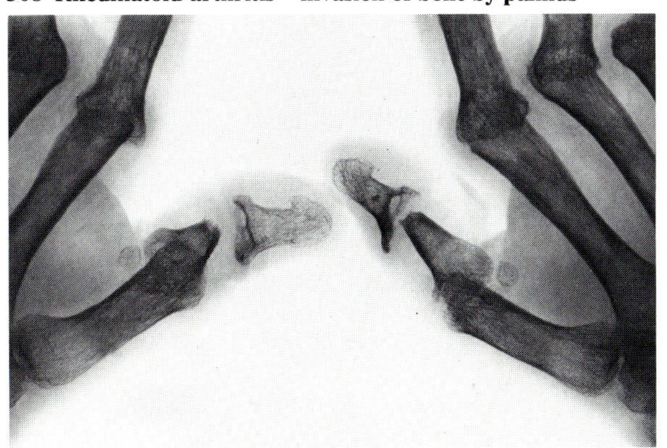

309 Rheumatoid arthritis – invasion of bone by pannus

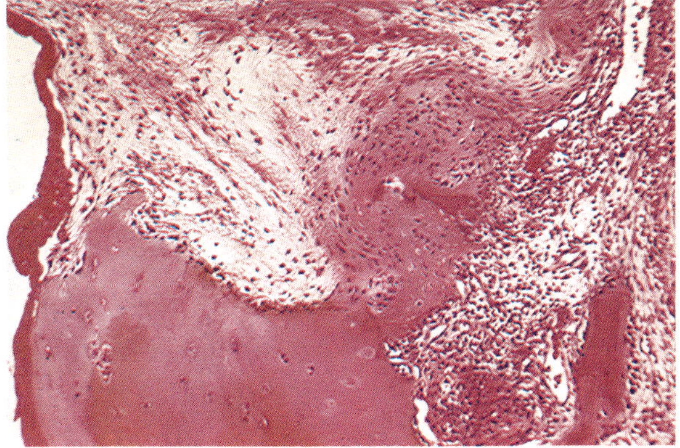

310 Rheumatoid arthritis

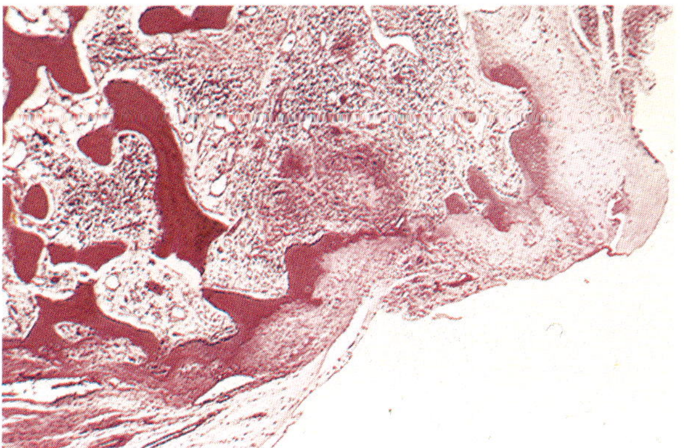

311 Osteo-arthrosis in knee joint

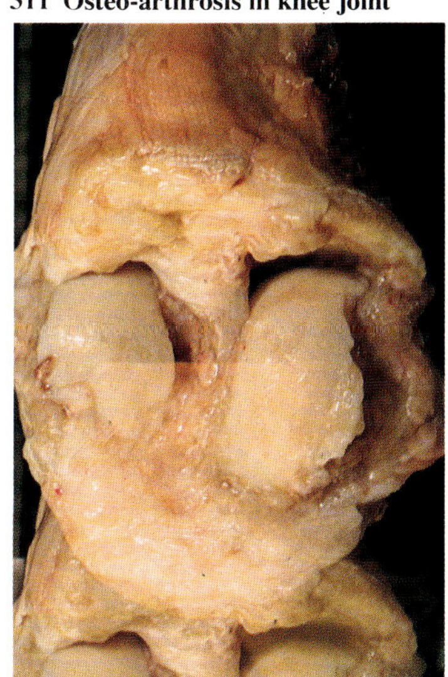

Extensions of synovial fluid to form bursae (**312**) and extensions into muscle have already been described (see **46**).

Clinically there is swelling around proximal joints in the hand and muscle wasting secondary to the inflammatory disease. This coupled with tendon involvement leads to the typical ulnar deviation in the hand (**313**).

In severely affected patients there is a collapse of bone and consequent shortening of the fingers which wobble insecurely on deformed metacarpels, 'arthritis mutilans' (**314**).

This extensive process in the cervical spine can cause atlanto-occipital joint destruction and the odontoid peg can impinge on the spinal cord leading to extensive neurological damage (**315**).

312 Rheumatoid bursa on elbow

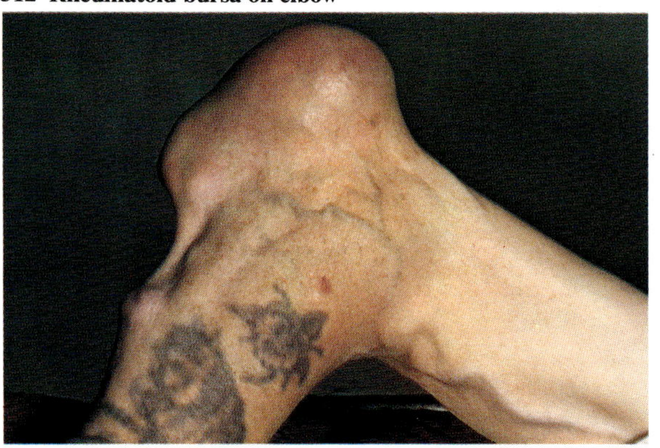

313 Rheumatoid joint deformities

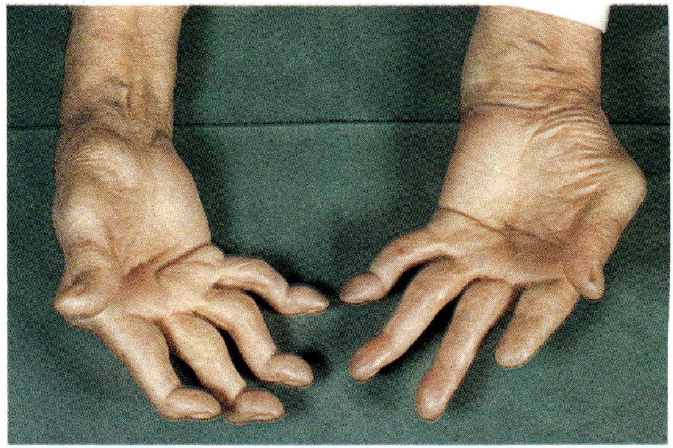

314 'Arthritis mutilans'

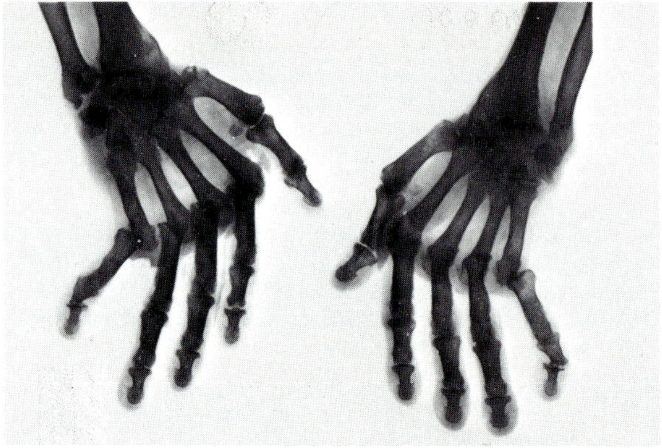

315 Rheumatoid spinal dislocation

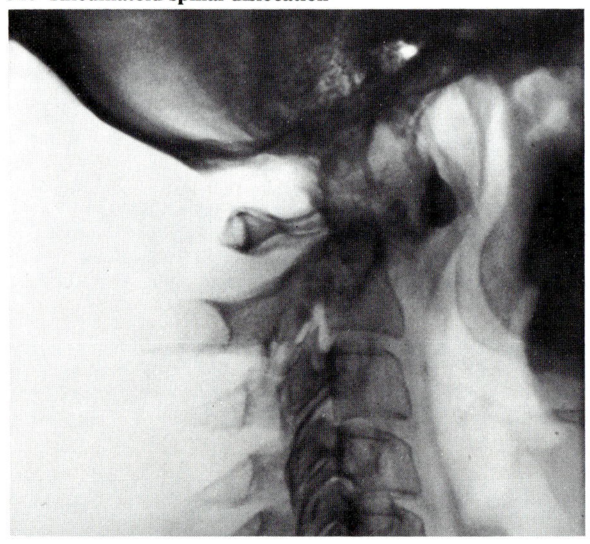

b. Psoriatic arthritis – inflammatory changes appear in the distal joints which are associated with skin changes and nail deformities (**316**).
c. Disseminated lupus, (DLE) Sjögrens syndrome, scleroderma (**317**) and mixed connective disease (a syndrome combining changes of DLE, scleroderma and rheumatoid-like changes), all give rise to joint changes which have the same appearance as rheumatoid arthritis.

316 Psoriatic arthritis

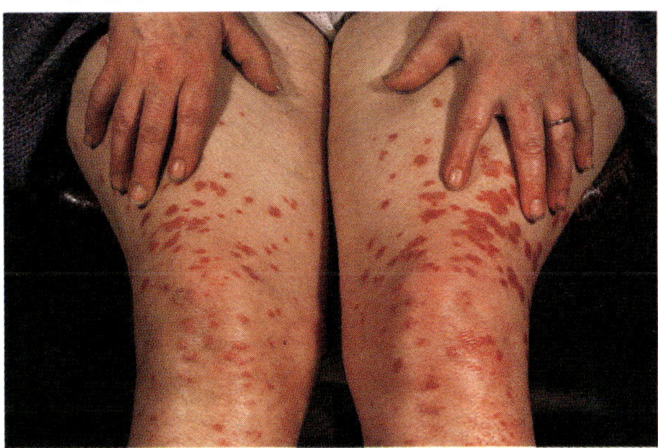

317 Scleroderma

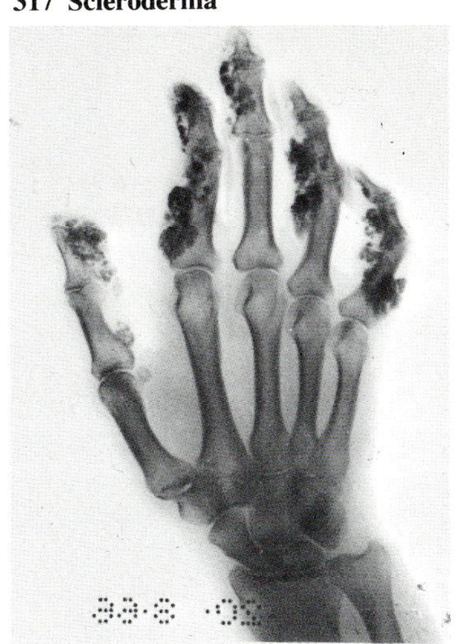

d. Juvenile rheumatoid arthritis (Still's disease) – when the bone is involved in the inflammatory process, various changes take place in maturation.

Changes in the hand include:

- retardation and irregularity of metatarsal growth
- premature closure of the epiphysis (**318**)
- irregularities of the joint surface
- dislocation of joint surfaces (**319**)

318 Still's disease

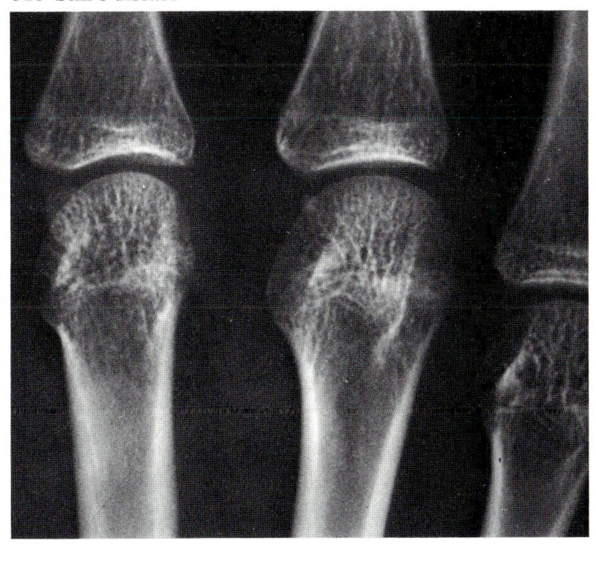

319 Still's disease

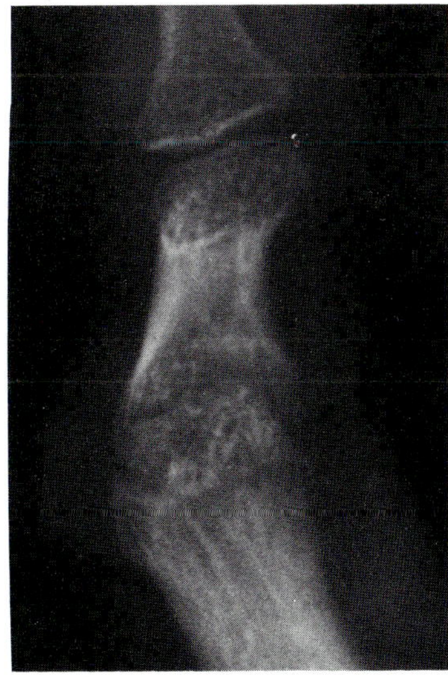

e. Rheumatic fever – rarely leads to joint deformities, but they may occasionally persist in the hands as Jocoud's arthritis causing spindling and flexion deformities in the fingers.

iv. Metabolic arthritis – primary metabolic rather than inflammatory or immunological changes are the cause of pain, effusions and limitation of movement. This does not rule out the activation of inflammatory mechanisms and complement activation as in acute gout. The common factor is the deposition of crystalline material due to supersaturation of the tissues or their failure to remove crystals by solution and phagocytosis.

a. Deposition of uric acid, gout. The deposition of uric acid occurs in the ears as tophi, around the joints as gouty arthritis (**320**) and within organs such as the kidney to cause a gouty nephropathy. Neat punched out holes occur in bone near the joint margins and more rarely extend into the joint space. On section birefringent crystals within the bone marrow with inflammatory cells near the periphery of the crystal mass can be seen.

b. Deposition of pyrophosphate crystals, 'pseudogout'. The collection of these crystals in the joint cartilage and in leucocytes (**321**) is followed by effusions into the joint and synovial reaction (**322** *alizarin* × *60*) can be caused by:
   - hypophosphatasia – failure to remove pyrophosphate (PP)
   - hyperparathyroidism – ? influx of PP in tissues
   - haemosiderosis – iron deposition blocking PP enzymes
   - heavy metal toxins, e.g. Cd

   Chronic chondrocalcinosis (**323**) leads to a break up of the cartilage and eventual destructive eburnation of bone with microfracture of the underlying trabeculae.

c. Deposition of hydroxyapatite crystals, e.g. acute polyosteoarthritis. Examination of synovial fluid from acute arthritic joints shows the presence of wear and tear particles of mineral crystals which may originate in matrix vesicles. Their liberation is associated with synovial inflammatory changes, migration of leucocytes and proliferation of chondrocytes. Acrylic fragments associated with phagocytosis by leucocytes can occasionally be found in the synovial fluid of joints with acrylic protheses.

d. Alkaptonuria – this inherited enzyme deficiency leads to an advanced arthropathy of the spine and hips with crystalline deposits of homogentisic acids seen in the vertebral discs (**324**), and a severe arthropathy in the hips (**325**).

e. Hyperparathyroidism – periosteal erosions near the joint consisting of osteoclastic proliferation and bone destruction (**326** *demineralised section, H&E* × *280*) lead to a painful destructive arthritis as seen in the acromioclavicular joint of a patient with 3° hyperparathyroidism (**327**).

320 Gouty arthritis

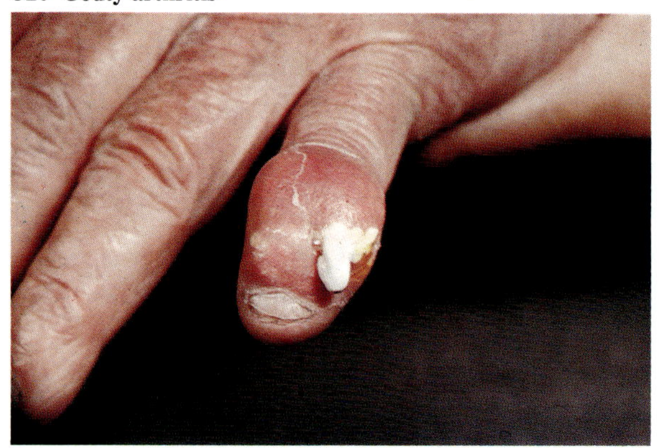

321 Pseudogout – crystal

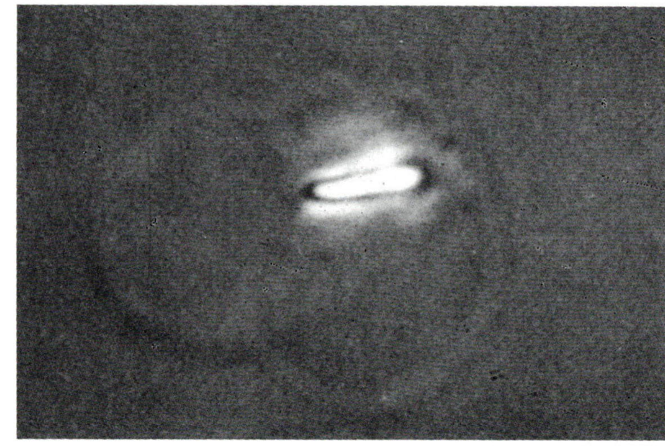

322 Pseudogout – crystal arthropathy

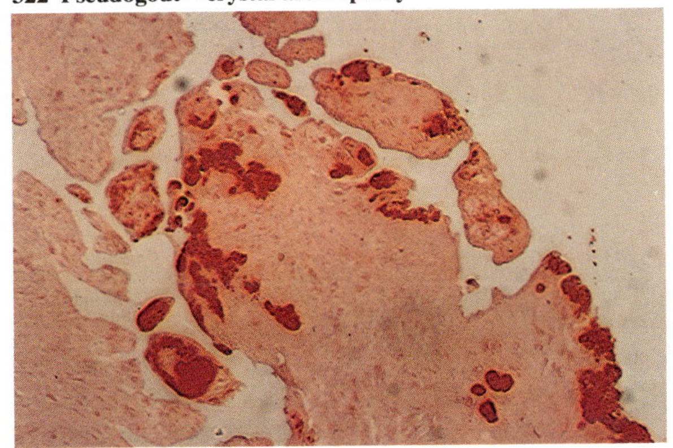

323 Chronic chondrocalcinosis

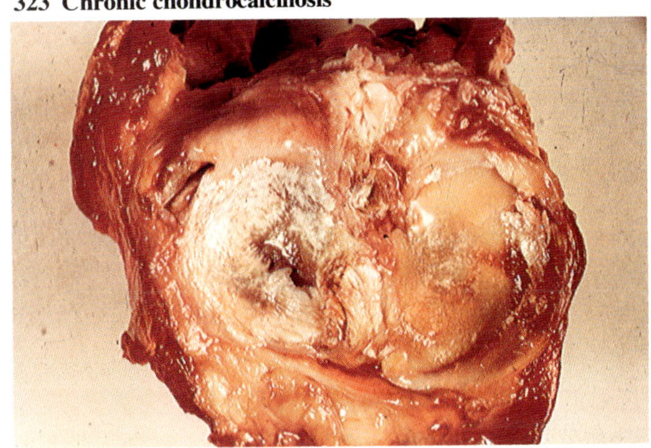

324 Alkaptonuric spine

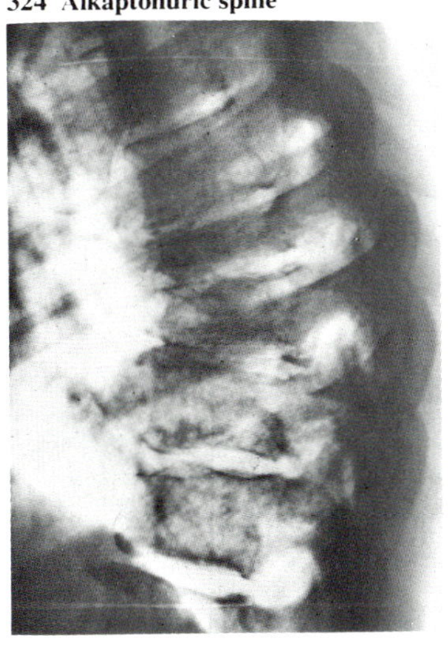

325 Alkaptonuric arthropathy

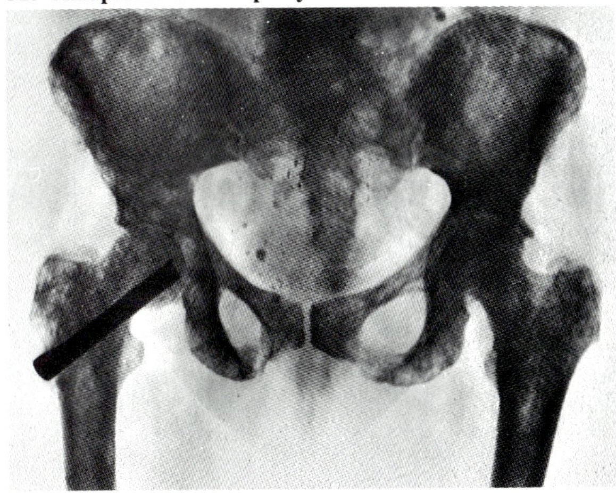

326 Hyperparathyroidism – bone erosion

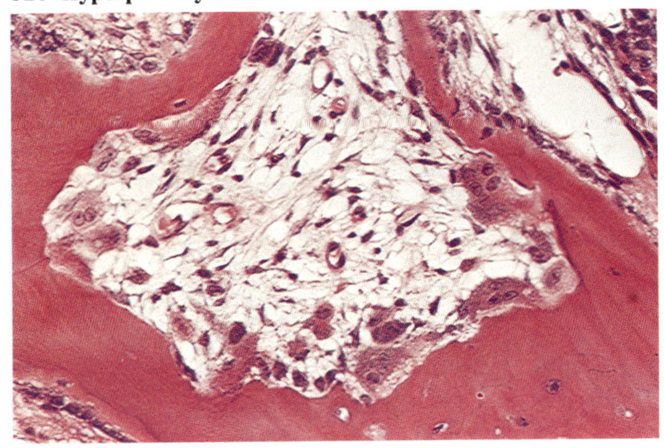

327 Hyperparathyroidism – acromioclavicular joint destruction

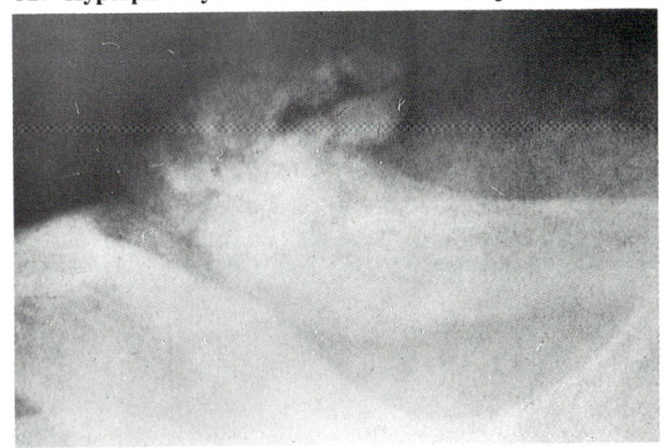

v. Neuropathic or Charcot joints – denervation leads to excessive wear on the cartilage joint surfaces, destruction of bone, instability of the joint and osteophyte formation (**328**). Causes include diabetes, neurosyphilis, leprosy, syringomyelia and haemophilia (**329**).

328 Charcot joint – knee

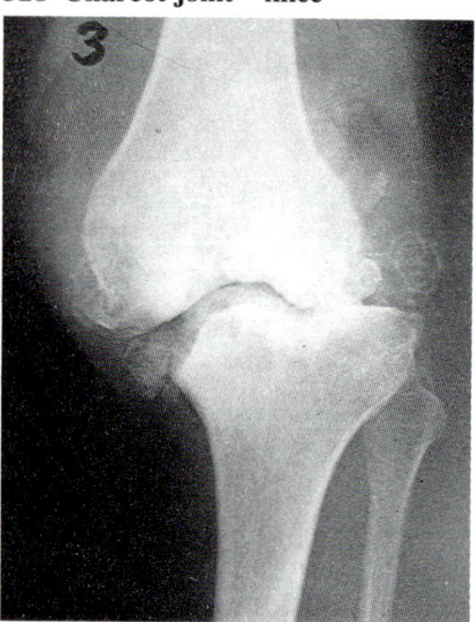

329 Haemophilia – knee joint

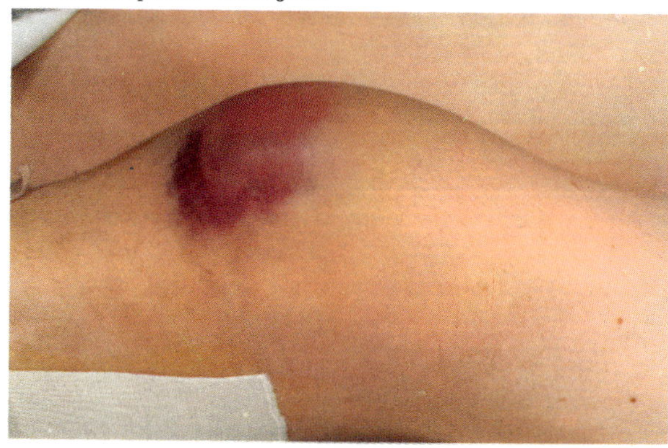

vi. Malignant disease – although some changes may be due to immune deposits provoking a synovial reaction, the majority involve malignant cells destroying bone and invading the joint from the bone. The synovial effusions are often blood-stained and may contain bony fragments.

An extremely rare form of arthritis most commonly seen in carcinoma of the bronchus takes the form of an acute periosteal reaction which can involve the synovia: acute pulmonary osteoarthropathy. The periosteum is seen lifted off the bone on radiological examination (**330**).

330 Periosteal elevation in carcinoma of bronchus

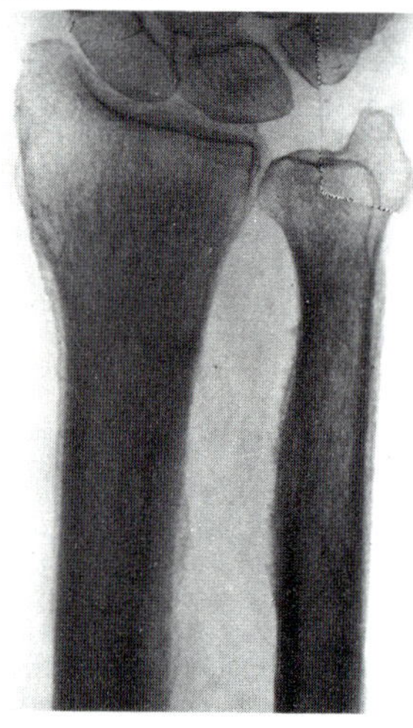

5. Dysplasia in the epiphyses and metaphyses

Many of the diseases already discussed may affect epiphyseal development and produce stunting of bone growth, deformity and degenerative changes in nearly all joints. They include achondroplasia, Gaucher's disease and osteogenesis imperfecta all of which may appear at birth and infancy and lead to dwarfism, pathological fracture and severe disability. The remaining group of diseases is frequently being added to and classification is complex. Inheritance is common and expert advice is available for the afflicted family from a few specialised centres where family inheritance is being classified.

One approach to classification is according to the site of the disorganised development which may be a hypoplasia or hyperplasia. Irregular processes of epiphyseal growth allow classification into those which occur in the epiphysis, the metaphysis and the diaphysis, the latter involving the shaft of the bone and endosteum.

Finally, the pathology varies from arrested to hyperplastic growth in the epiphyseal cartilage and its various layers near the epiphysis and the epiphyseal plate. This causes continued abnormalities of modelling of the shaft and epiphysis leading to altered density and irregular masses of cartilage and bone (**331** and **332**). Contractures around joints and exostoses are common. The irregularity may give rise to the possible diagnosis of malignancy.

Other connective tissue changes are seen in the eye, skin and kidney. Skull deformities lead to hydrocephalus, chest abnormalities to respiratory failure and renal disease accompanies some forms of skeletal dwarfism. Polydactyly and heart lesions are occasionally linked with these abnormalities.

331 Bone dysplasia – classification

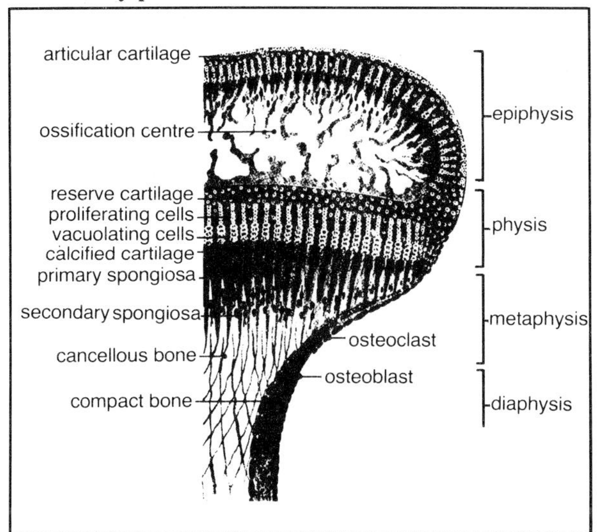

332 Bone dysplasia – classification

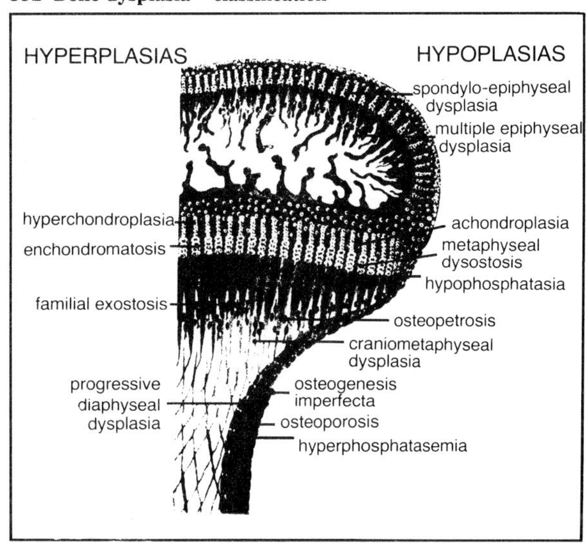

6. Inflammatory disease of bone

a. Osteomyelitis

Osteomyelitis is inflammation of the bone and bone marrow due to bacterial infection. Acute osteomyelitis is seen most frequently in children but may occur at any age. Micro-organisms may reach bone via the blood-stream and by direct innoculation from the body surface as in a compound fracture. Blood-borne infection, especially by Staphylococcus aureus which is often penicillin resistant, is the commonest cause.

Aspiration of the lesion is generally necessary to confirm the diagnosis, identify the organism and ascertain its antibiotic sensitivity, and to relieve pressure.

The common site is the metaphyseal end of a long bone. If the infection is not aborted by prompt antibiotic treatment the infected bone will become rarefied, the surrounding bone will show sclerosis and periosteal new bone formation will occur (**333**).

Chronic osteomyelitis of the calcaneum (**334**). The bone is destroyed and a sinus opens onto the skin of the posterior part of the heel. The marrow space is occupied by pus and granulation tissue (**335** *H&E × 350*). The pressure of the exudate in the unyielding bone causes bone necrosis.

333 Osteomyelitis – rarefaction and sclerosis of bone

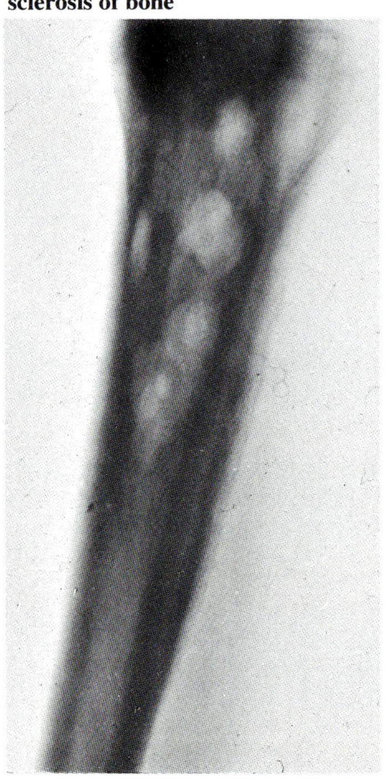

334 Osteomyelitis – calcaneum

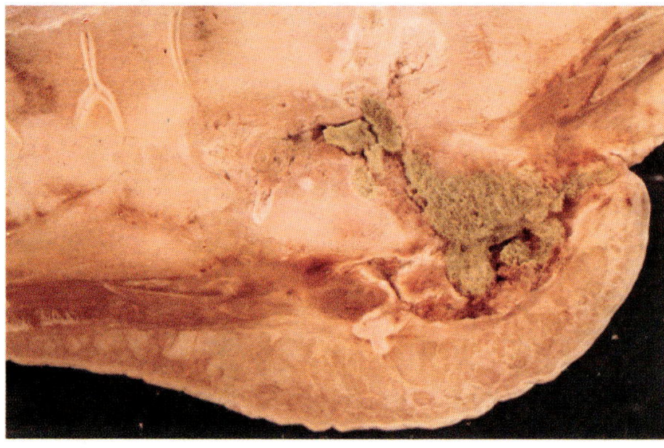

335 Osteomyelitis – pus and granulation tissue

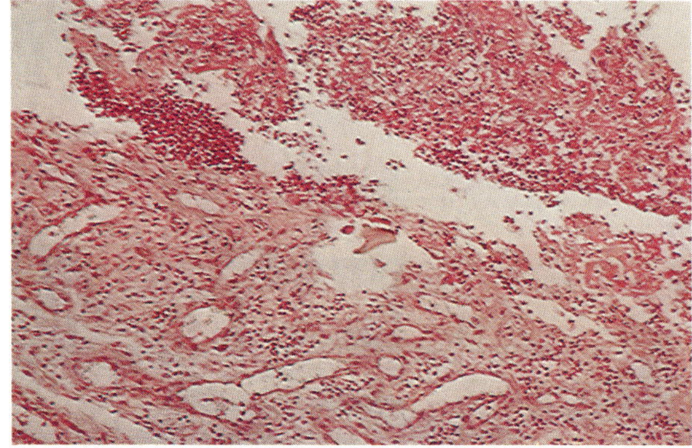

A sinus discharging pus from osteomyelitis onto the skin (**336**). The infection first spreads through the haversian canals of the bone to the marrow cavity and then to the sub-periosteal region. The periosteum is sometimes stripped from the bone. The new bone which forms beneath the elevated periosteum is known as an involucrum.

Necrotic bone separates from viable bone to form a sequestrum, and if not too large may be extruded through a sinus. Very small sequestra are resorbed by osteoclasts. Note the loss of osteocytes from the lacunae indicating death of the bone (**337** *demineralised section, H&E × 350*).

In the spine a central cavity extending across a disc space is characteristic of a bone abscess (**338**) which shows up as an area of increased uptake on a Sr^{85} scan (**339**).

336 Osteomyelitis – sinus formation

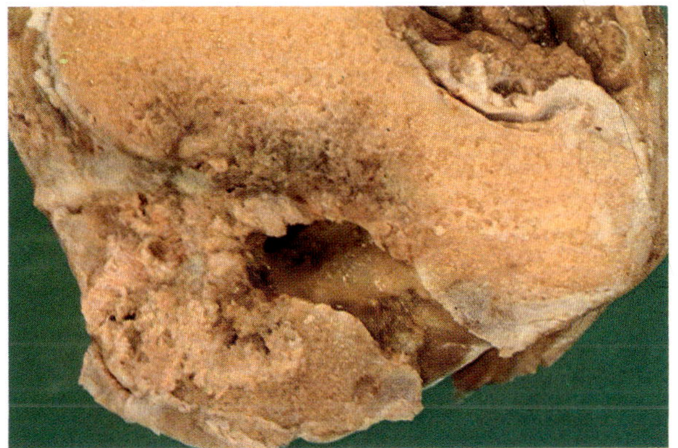

337 Osteomyelitis – sequestrum

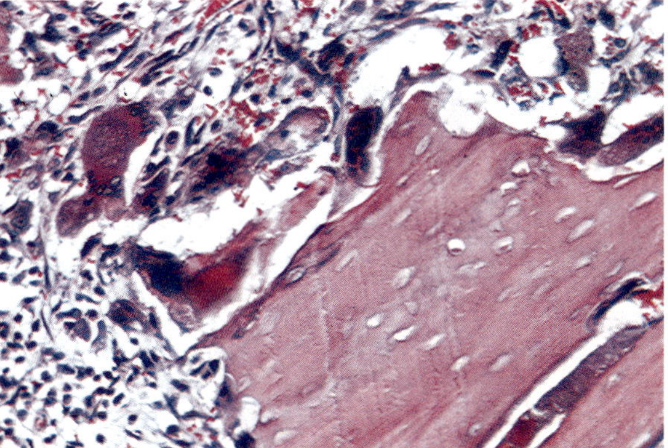

338 Osteomyelitis of spine

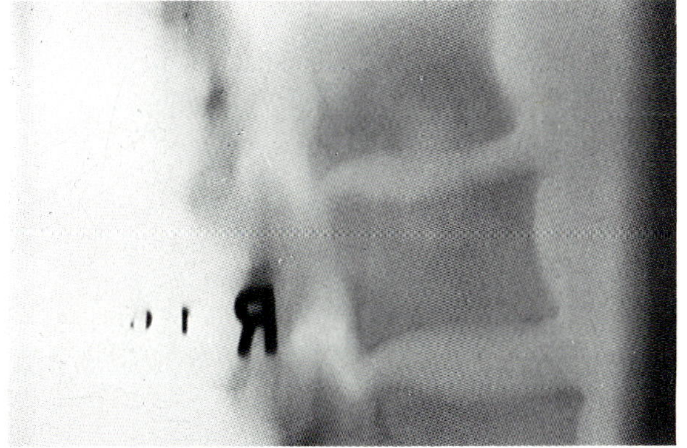

339 Osteomyelitis of spine – vertebral abscess

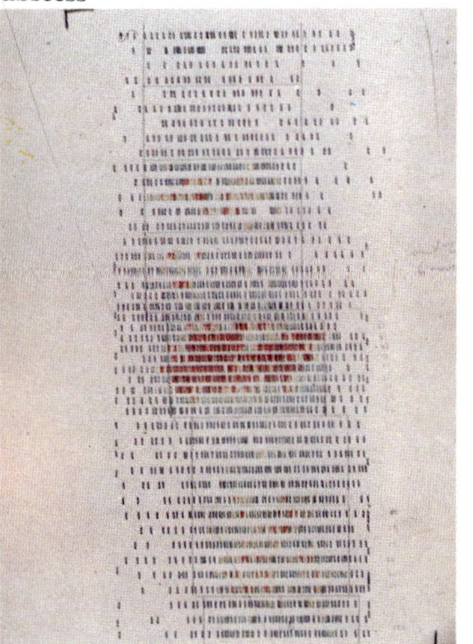

Among the less common blood-borne infections are those due to salmonella organisms. These tend to give rise to multiple foci of infection. Salmonella osteomyelitis is a complication of sickle cell anaemia. A combination of bone marrow thrombosis and infarction plus the decreased ability of macrophages to phagocytose bacteria as a result of engorgement of reticulo-endothelial cells with red blood cells may be involved. But this does not explain the unique susceptibility of patients with sickle cell disease to bone infection by salmonella organisms. The bone marrow hyperplasia associated with sickle cell disease is seen in **340** in the skull and sternum. Radiological changes in the tibiae of a young boy with salmonella osteomyelitis are shown in **341**.

A rare complication of chronic suppurative osteomyelitis is squamous cell carcinoma developing in sinuses draining the lesion. The carcinoma, first described by Marjolin, usually presents as a fungating, malodorous mass with a coating of exudate (**342**). Most of these squamous carcinomas are well differentiated, however in spite of resection or amputation they metastasize and kill the patient. A second rare complication is amyloidosis. Chronic osteomyelitis is a declining cause of amyloidosis, but as in other cases of chronic suppuration, the patient is at risk of developing this disease.

In adults osteomyelitis can be a chronic disease of insidious onset, difficult to distinguish clinically and radiologically from primary or metastatic malignancy; a bone biopsy is usually necessary.

A section shows little or no pus, instead a chronic inflammatory cell infiltrate, granulation tissue formation and fibrous and reactive bone formation are visible (**343** *demineralised section, H&E × 50*).

340 Sickle cell disease – bone marrow hyperplasia

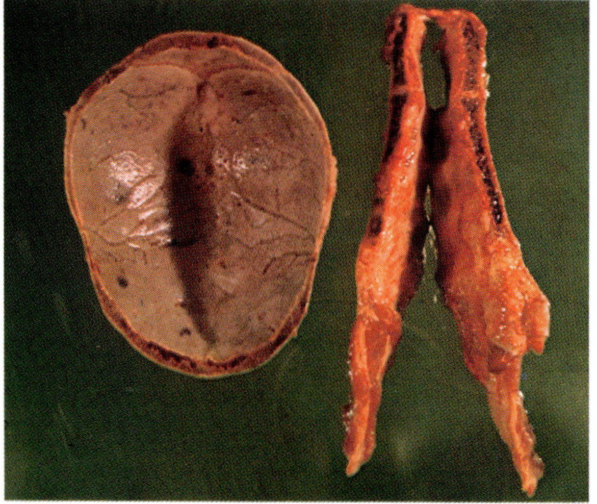

341 Salmonella osteomyelitis

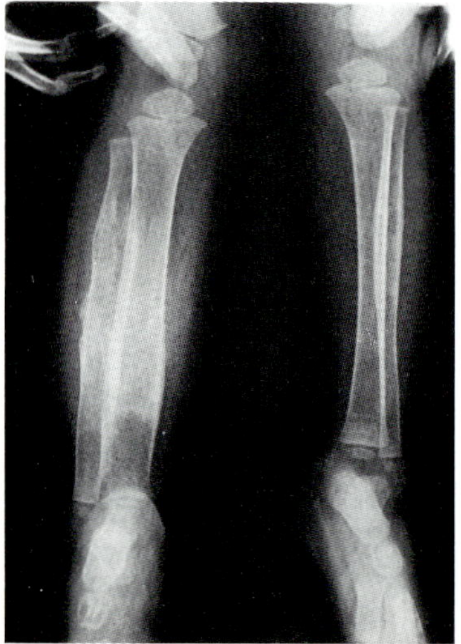

342 Squamous cell carcinoma complicating osteomyelitis

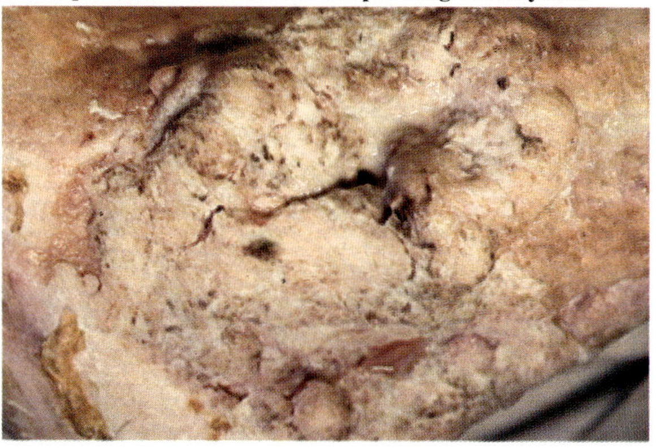

343 Chronic osteomyelitis

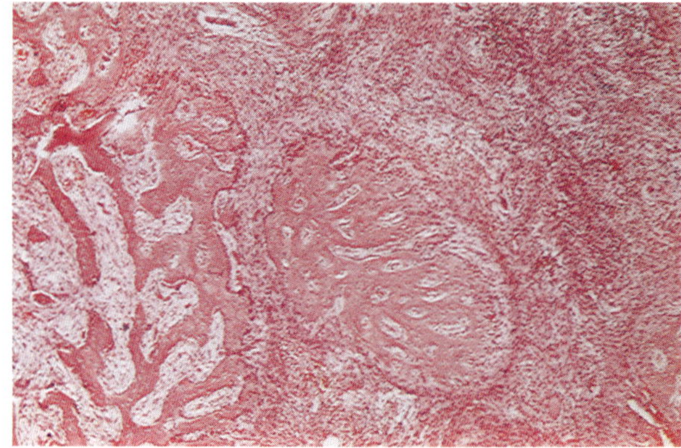

b. Tuberculosis

In tuberculous osteomyelitis a plain X-ray reveals rarefaction, 'cold abscess' formation and destruction of bone and occasionally calcified 'cold abscess' formation beyond the bone. A young patient with tuberculosis of the spine (**344**).

The typical angular kyphosis of Pott's disease of the lower thoracic vertebrae is seen in **345**. The disease starts in the trabecular bone of the vertebral body and eventually the intervertebral disc is eroded and adjacent vertebrae are involved. Anterior collapse of a single or adjacent vertebrae causes the angulation of the spine shown here.

The spine is the commonest site of bone involvement and accounts for 50 per cent of cases of tuberculous osteomyelitis. The thoracic, lumbar and cervical vertebrae are involved in that order of frequency. The complications of Pott's disease are 'cold abscess' formation, paraplegia and nerve root compression, osteoarthrosis and amyloidosis. Paraplegia is the result of pressure on the cord by tuberculous tissue or collapsed vertebrae.

The basic lesion is the tubercle consisting of a central caseous area surrounded by epithelioid cells and Langhans' giant cells with an outer zone of lymphocytes. The proliferation of tubercles and their confluence results in bone destruction (**346** *demineralised section, H&E × 250*).

344 Tuberculous osteomyelitis of spine

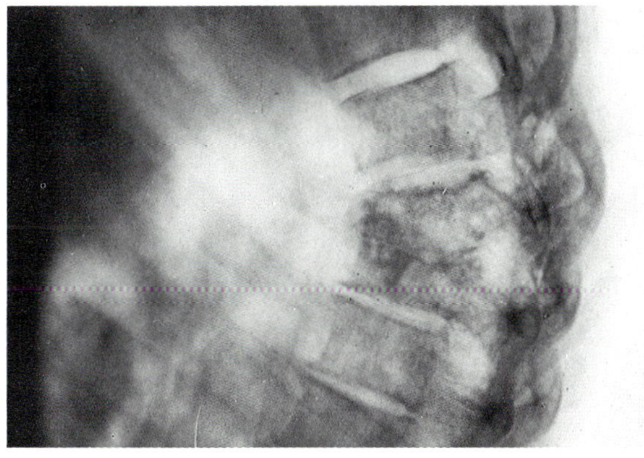

346 Tuberculous osteomyelitis

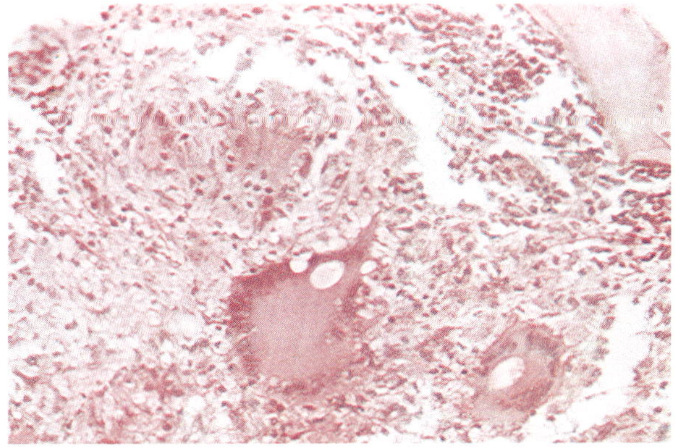

345 Pott's disease of spine

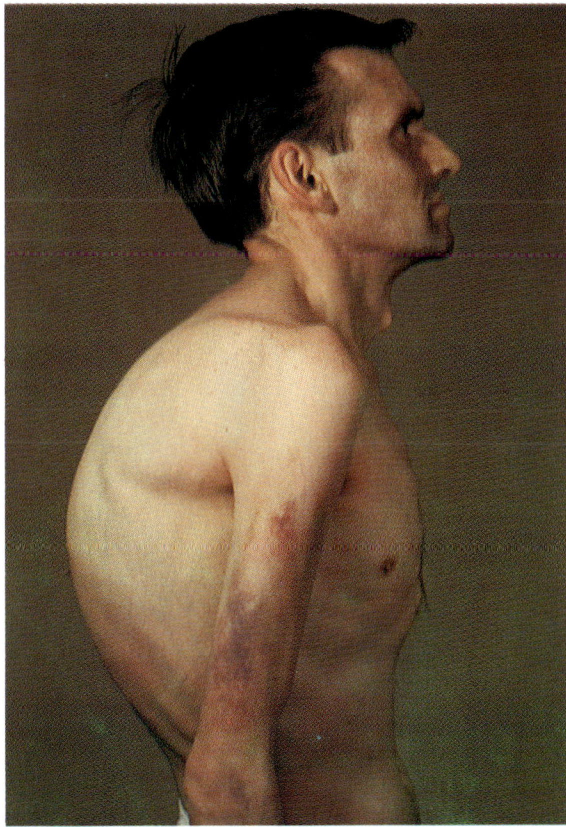

Deposits of amyloid in the spleen of a patient with tuberculous osteomyelitis (**347** × *180*). The presence of amyloid, stained by Congo red and viewed with the polarizing microscope, is confirmed by its green yellow birefringence.

347 Amyloidosis complicating tuberculous osteomyelitis

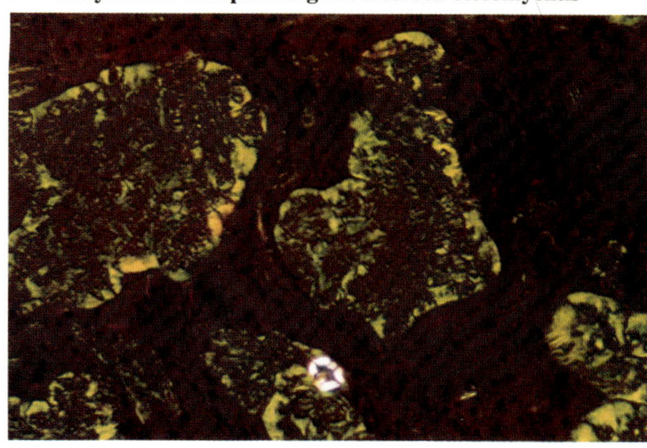

c. Leprosy

The disease produces skin ulceration, loss of tissue including bone; terminal digit erosions are shown in **348**. Further Charcot-like changes around joints occur secondary to the peripheral neuropathy.

348 Leprosy – phalangeal destruction

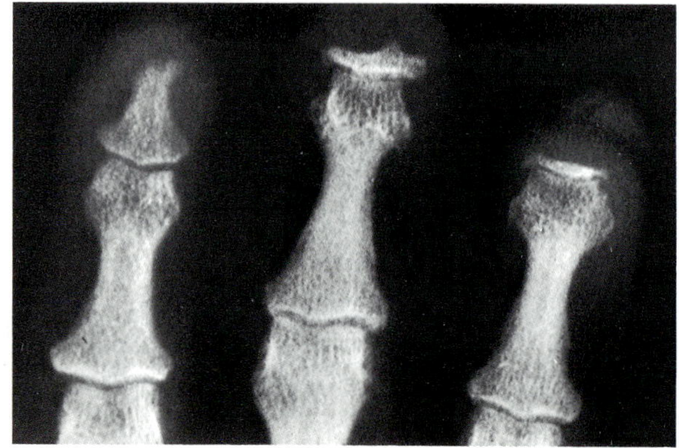

d. Syphilis

Bone lesions in syphilis are seen only rarely. They may be congenital or acquired.

Congenital syphilis of bone is encountered most frequently in the form of epiphysitis in which the epiphyseal plate is thickened or replaced by a zone of granulation tissue and fibrous tissue. The lesion teems with Treponemas. The complications are retardation of bone formation and separation of the epiphyses, both of which interfere with growth. Disease of the nasal bones results in destruction of the nasal septum and a 'saddle nose' (**349**). Defective dentition is manifest as peg-shaped, notched incisor teeth referred to as Hutchinson's teeth (**350**).

In acquired syphilis gumma formation is usually associated with periostitis, these being the two most common lesions. Gummas may destroy bone and discharge by a sinus on to the skin especially if complicated by secondary infection. In the skull a large area of bone may be destroyed and the dura exposed. The combination of bone destruction and heaped up, thickened, irregular, bony margins is typical of a gummatous lesion (**351**). In the palate, gummatous periositis causes ulceration followed by perforation of the hard palate (**352** and **353**) and nasal septum.

349 Congenital syphilis – saddle nose

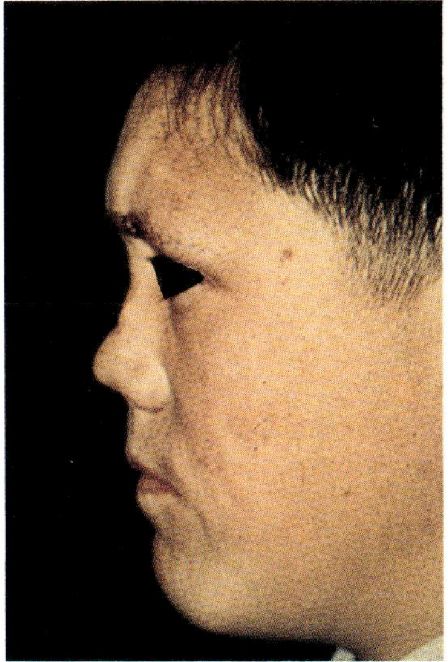

350 Congenital syphilis – Hutchinson's teeth

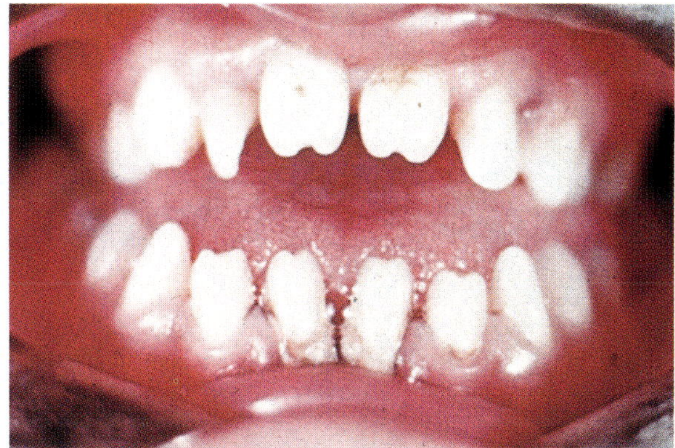

351 Syphilis – destruction of skull by gumma

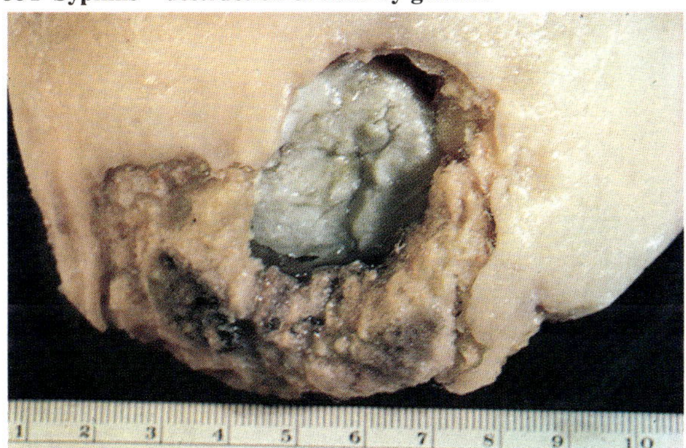

352 Syphilis – bone destruction by gumma

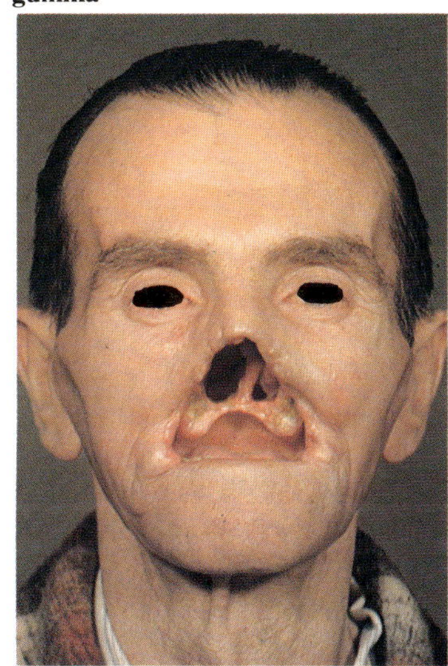

353 Syphilis – perforation of hard palate and nasal septum

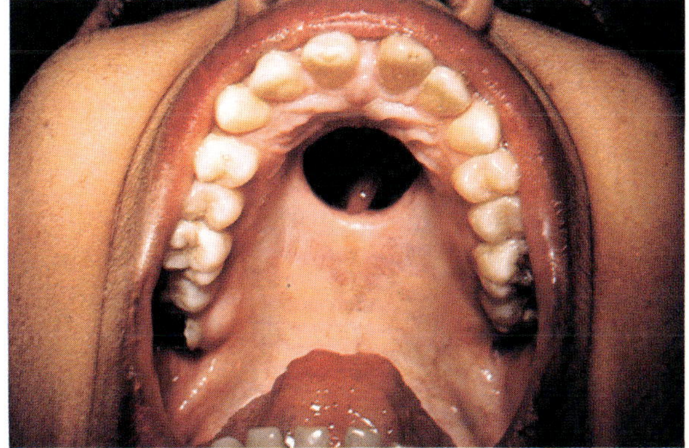

Appendix

The foods below are referred to in the tables on page 10, 100 g portions are illustrated.

354 Calcium content

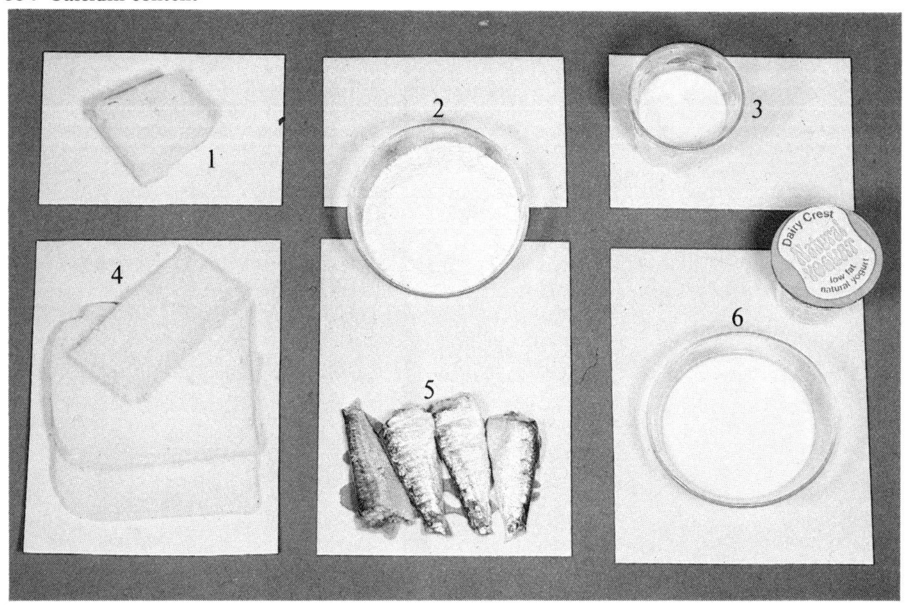

1 – cheese
2 – dried potato
3 – milk
4 – white bread
5 – sardines
6 – skimmed milk

355 Phosphate content

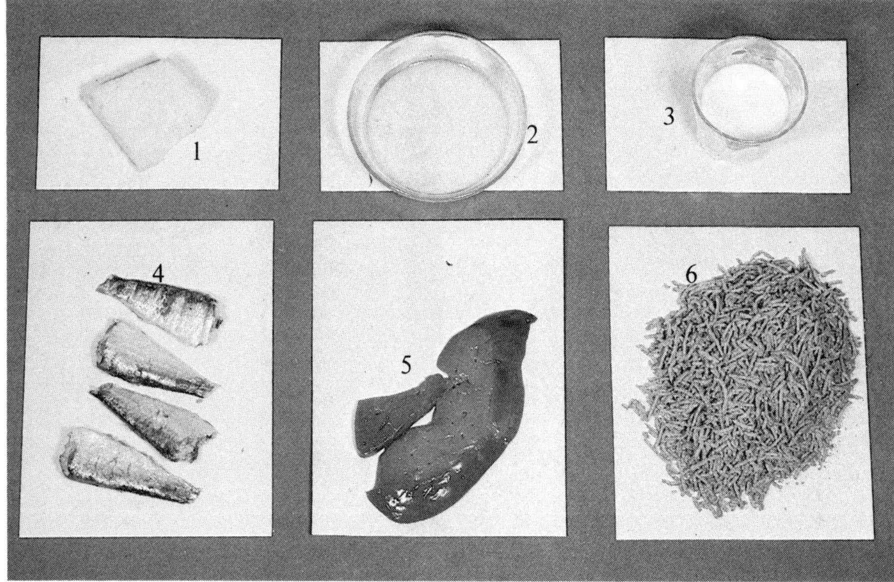

1 – cheese
2 – egg yolks
3 – dried milk
4 – sardines
5 – liver
6 – bran

356 Vitamin D content

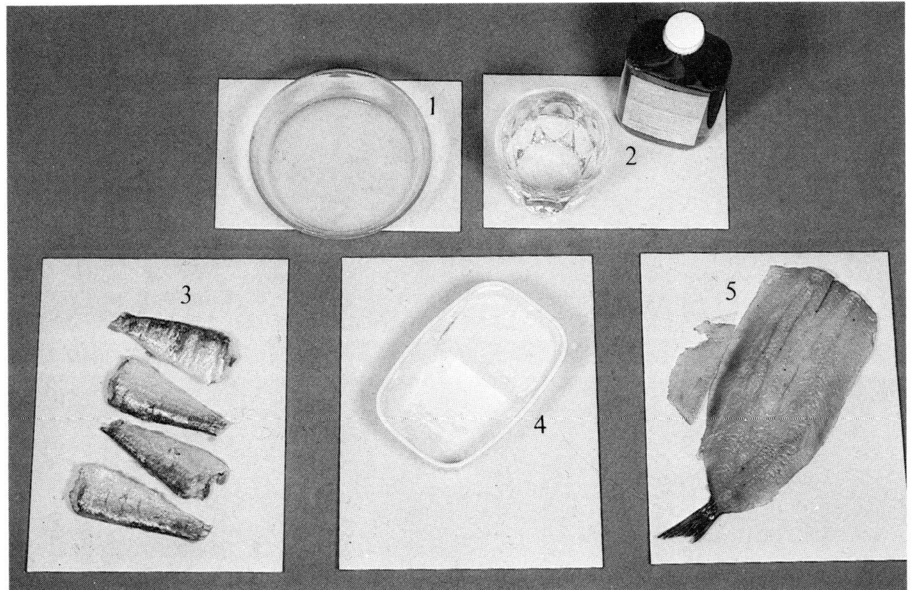

1 – milk
2 – cod liver oil
3 – sardines
4 – margarine
5 – raw kippers

357 Vitamin C content

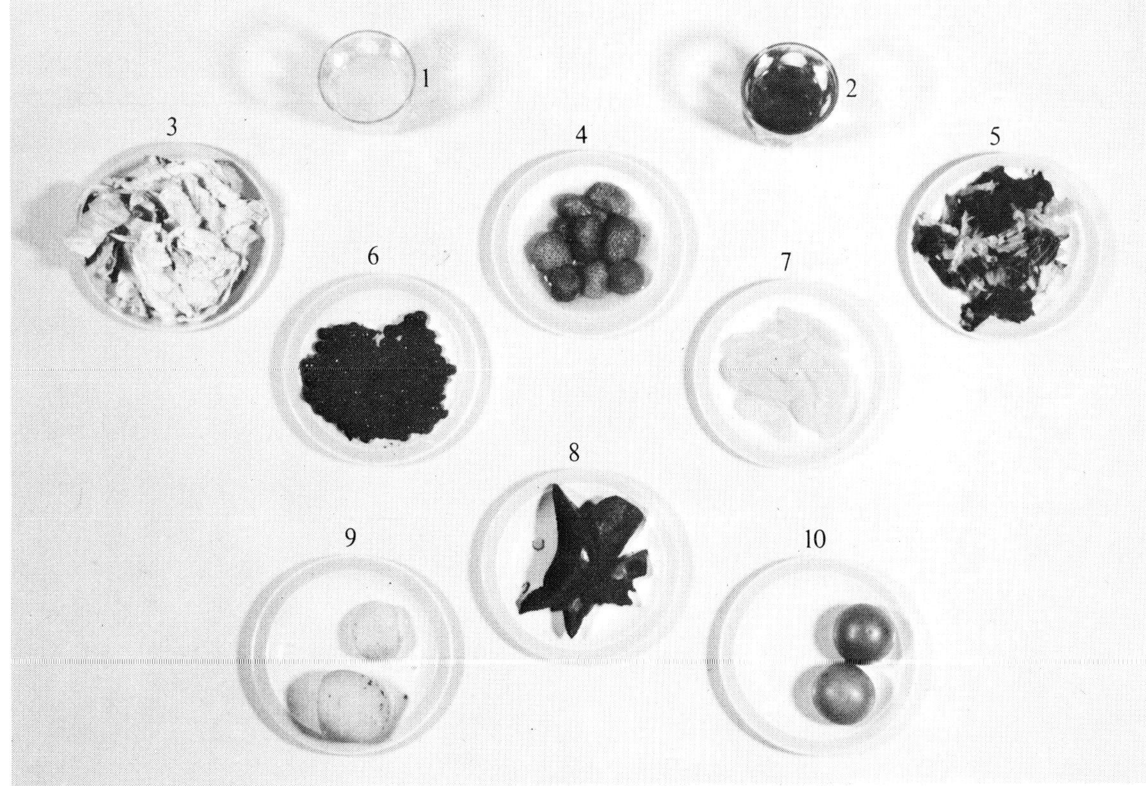

1 – grapefruit juice
2 – rose hip syrup
3 – raw cabbage
4 – fresh strawberries
5 – cooked cabbage
6 – blackcurrants
7 – oranges
8 – fried liver
9 – new potatoes
10 – tomatoes

Bibliography

Avioli, L. V. and Krane, S. M. (Eds.) (1977). *Metabolic Bone Disease*. Vols. I and II. Academic Press Inc., London.

Barry, H. C. (1969). *Paget's Disease of Bone*. E. & S. Livingstone Ltd.

Bickel, H. and Stern, J. (Eds.) (1976). *Inborn Errors of Calcium and Bone Metabolism*. Proc. XIIth Symposium of Society of Inborn Errors of Metabolism, MTP Press Ltd.

Dahlin, D. C. (1974). *Bone Tumours*. C. Thomas Publishers.

Dequeker, J. (1972). *Bone Loss in Normal and Pathological Conditions*. Leuven University Press.

Fourman, P. and Royer, P. (1968). *Calcium Metabolism and the Bone*. 2nd edn. Blackwell Scientific Publications.

Jowsey, J. (1977). *Metabolic Diseases of Bone*. Vol. I in series. W. B. Saunders Co.

Nordin, B. E. C. (Ed.) (1976). *Calcium Phosphate and Magnesium Metabolism*. Churchill Livingstone.

Paterson, C. R. (1974). *Metabolic Disorders of Bone*. Blackwell Scientific Publications.

Rasmussen, H. and Bordier, P. (1974). *The Physiological and Cellular Basis of Metabolic Bone Diseases*. The Williams and Wilkins Co., Baltimore.

Rubin, P. (1964). *Bone Dysplasias – A Dynamic Approach*. Year Book Medical Publications, Chicago.

Smith, R. (1979). *Biochemical Disorders of the Skeleton*. Postgraduate Orthopaedics Series, Ed. A. Graham Apley. Butterworths.

Spanger, J. W., Langer, L. O. and Wiedemann, H. R. (1974). *Bone Dysplasias – An Atlas of Constitutional Disorders of Skeletal Development*. W. B. Saunders Co., Philadelphia.

Vaughan, J. M. (1975). *The Physiology of Bone*. 2nd edn. Clarendon Press.

Wynne-Davies, R. and Fairbank, T. J. (1976). *Fairbank's Atlas of General Affections of the Skeleton*. 2nd edn. Churchill Livingstone.

Index

(Numbers in bold type refer to illustrations.)

Index

(Numbers in bold type refer to illustrations.)